Happy
HORMONES

Happy
HORMONES

Discover the Breakthrough Treatment Program
for Better Hormonal Health

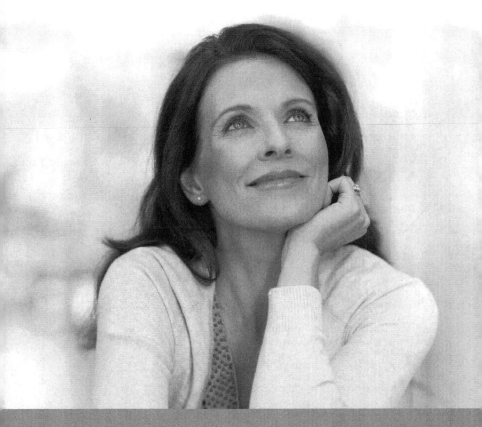

Natural Treatment Programs for:
Weight Loss • PMS • Menopause • Fatigue • Irritability

KRISTY VERMEULEN, ND
FOREWORD BY DIRK VAN LITH, MD

))) hatherleigh

Happy Hormones

Text Copyright © 2014 Kristy Vermeulen

Library of Congress Cataloging-in-Publication Data is available.

ISBN: 978-1-57826-486-5

Cover Design by Chris Sheesley
Interior & Back Cover Design by Carolyn Kasper

Printed in the United States

10 9 8 7 6 5 4

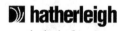

www.hatherleighpress.com

Dedication

To the millions of women suffering from hormonal imbalances who have been told there is nothing wrong and that their symptoms are normal.

To all the health-care practitioners who are reading this book because they want to better understand how they can help their patients balance their hormones.

And to my family and my amazing husband Jasper for your unconditional love and support.

—*Kristy Vermeulen, ND*

Contents

PART 4
PUTTING IT ALL TOGETHER

PART 5
APPENDIX

PART 6
HAPPY HORMONES RECIPE COLLECTION

Foreword

MILLIONS OF women suffer from hormonal imbalances, such as difficulty losing weight, fatigue, irritability, and brain fog, yet these imbalances are often overlooked and untreated. Dr. Kristy Vermeulen's *Happy Hormones* offers a revolutionary breakthrough in understanding the most common hormonal imbalances, along with how best to support the women who are dealing with these imbalances.

Dr. Kristy uses a fascinating approach, combining both allopathic and integrative medicine in her *Happy Hormones* diagnosis and treatment programs. By bringing together her clinical experience, naturopathic medical training, and the latest research, she was able to provide a comprehensive guide to help women effectively assess and treat the most common hormonal imbalances. As I read through this book, I am continually impressed with Dr. Kristy's ability to clarify and simplify the complex world of hormones.

The book begins with Dr. Kristy explaining what exactly hormones are, and why they are so important to our health and well-being. She continues on to describe, simply and clearly, the most frequently seen hormonal imbalances—cortisol, thyroid, estrogen, progesterone, testosterone, and DHEA excesses and deficiencies are all expertly discussed, along with how these imbalances affect us. Using a comprehensive questionnaire, accompanied by symptom tables and suggested laboratory tests, Dr. Kristy further outlines how to identify these six common sources of hormonal imbalances. By understanding which hormonal imbalances are directly affecting your health, you can immediately begin to make the changes necessary to balance your levels and reclaim your energy, mood, and overall health.

For me, the highlight of the book are the Happy Hormones treatment programs. In these chapters, Dr. Kristy takes the time to go into greater detail regarding each of the potential hormonal excesses and deficiencies, providing nutritional and lifestyle guidance, along with specific herbal, vitamin, and bioidentical hormone recommendations for each imbalance. I found the treatment recommendations for adrenal fatigue and low thyroid function particularly interesting.

Over the years, I have seen Dr. Kristy's success in treating these imbalances in the faces of numerous grateful patients, one of whom was my own wife, whom she treated for adrenal fatigue. I have even incorporated some of Dr. Kristy's treatment suggestions for adrenal and thyroid imbalances into my own practice, with great success. It has been amazing to see the progress my patients make after addressing their hormonal imbalances: they lose weight more easily, their mood and energy levels improve, and they even sleep better.

By reading this book, practitioners and patients alike will learn how to connect the dots; determining the connections between vague symptoms such as fatigue, irritability, brain fog, difficulty losing weight, and menopause, and allowing them to make educated decisions for resolving particular hormonal imbalances. When these connections have been established, and any imbalances properly addressed, many women's lives will be changed for the better.

Happy Hormones offers newfound health to those who have been suffering with hormonal problems for much too long. It is a must-read for all women, especially if they are feeling fatigued, heavy, irritable, or menopausal.

—Dr. Dirk van Lith, MD, MPH, DTM&H,
author of *The Original European HCG Cure*

Introduction

Optimal hormone balance is necessary to live a life full of energy, health, and happiness. As a female naturopathic doctor who has been through her own hormonal imbalances, I have always searched for natural, safe solutions for balancing hormones. For years I suffered from high cortisol, then low cortisol, followed by estrogen excess and progesterone deficiency. Through these imbalances I experienced symptoms ranging from anxiety, PMS, eczema, menstrual cramps, low libido, and fatigue. But with the combination of research and years of experience, I created a treatment program that allowed me to break through those hormonal imbalances and regain my energy, concentration, and sex drive and say good-bye to the emotional roller-coaster that is PMS. I am so thankful that I discovered these solutions and I can't wait for you to discover them as well.

I have written this book for all the women out there suffering from hormonal imbalances, whether it is low energy, irritability, PMS, menstrual cramps, hot flashes, insomnia, low sex drive, weight gain, or infertility. I'm sure that, like many of my patients, you have most likely been to your doctor expressing some of these symptoms and been told it's nothing and that these symptoms are normal. But this is not true. Though these symptoms may be common, they are not normal. By acknowledging these symptoms and working to balance their hormones, I help women regain their vitality, energy, and health so they can live the healthy, fabulous life they deserve. It is my goal with this book to get you there as well.

Happy Hormones is a step-by-step guide to get your hormones back on track. It is designed to give you all the necessary information you need so you can assess your specific hormonal imbalance and successfully treat it through diet and lifestyle recommendations, nutritional supplements, homeopathic and herbal medicines, as well as bioidentical hormones. It is the same protocol that I have used in my practice to help hundreds of women attain optimal hormone balance, health, and happiness.

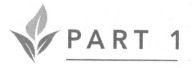

PART 1

Happy Hormones
Explained

CHAPTER 1

Dr. Kristy's Happy Hormones Program

MILLIONS OF women are living with hormonal imbalances every day without getting sufficient help. These imbalances can range from PMS, infertility, weight gain, and the terrible hot flashes experienced during menopause to fatigue, stress, anxiety, and poor memory. For years women have been searching for answers to help resolve these symptoms but they are often left feeling confused and hopeless after being told there is nothing that can be done. Fortunately there are many natural treatment options available to help you break through these imbalances and get back to the healthy, happy life you deserve. And it is this information I wish to share with you through the Happy Hormones program.

The Happy Hormones program helps you discover what your particular hormonal imbalances are so you can successfully treat them with a safe, scientifically based program. I've designed the program into four parts:

1. General information so you can better understand what hormones are and why they are important to your health

2. Hormone diagnosis, including a comprehensive questionnaire, symptom lists, and recommended lab testing to help you determine your particular hormone imbalances

3. A six-step hormone-balancing program to correct the hormonal imbalances and get you feeling healthy and fabulous again

4. A getting-started guide with a general nutrition program, recipes, and bioidentical hormone information to help you utilize the information in the best way possible

The Happy Hormones six-step balancing program is a comprehensive process, involving:

- Lifestyle modifications
- Dietary and nutritional changes
- Nutritional supplements
- Herbal support
- Homeopathic solutions
- Bioidentical hormone replacement therapy

Lifestyle and diet are considered the foundations of health. Without a solid, healthy foundation, many important bodily processes, such as detoxification, hormone production and metabolism, cognitive functioning, and energy production, are unable to properly function. We need these processes functioning at optimal levels to allow for successful results with the other steps in the Happy Hormones program.

Nutritional supplements are also an important part of the six-step treatment program. We require some very specific nutrients for hormone production and function. Depending on your particular hormonal imbalance, these can range from simple vitamins and minerals to homeopathics and ancient Indian herbs.

Bioidentical hormones are also included in the Happy Hormones treatment program. Some hormonal deficiencies, depending on the severity, respond faster with hormone supplementation. Because there is a lot of controversy around hormone replacement, I have included a separate chapter explaining the differences between synthetic and bioidentical hormones, as well as safe application and dosing methods.

By following this program, you will discover what your hormonal imbalances are and how to treat them in the most safe and effective way possible. *Happy Hormones* will help you regain your energy, vitality, and youth so you can live a healthy, fabulous life.

CHAPTER 2

What Are Hormones and Why Are They Important?

Why Hormones Are Important

Hormones are involved in almost every single process in our body. We need them to survive. Hormones manage our blood-sugar levels and weight, and support our immune system to help us better cope with stress and illness. Hormones give men "male" characteristics and women "female" characteristics. In women, they regulate the menstrual cycle, pregnancy, and birth, and in both men and women, they increase muscle and bone mass, confidence, and strength. Hormones also regulate our daily wake and sleep cycles and maintain our moods, energy, focus, and emotions.

As you can see, hormones are essential to life, especially for a life that is healthy and happy. Unfortunately, our bodies are not functioning with optimal hormonal levels these days. The environment we live in—with work stress, family stress, long hours, environmental pollution, inadequate sleep, and poor diet—is making it difficult for our bodies to produce optimal levels of these important hormones. We are constantly struggling just to make enough hormones to get us through the day. And if we are unable to produce optimal levels, hormonal-related symptoms can start to show up. These symptoms can range from anxiety and difficulty sleeping to hot flashes, weight gain, and infertility. It is important to address hormonal health and maintain optimal levels so you can live the healthy, energetic life you deserve.

What Are Hormones?

Hormones are biological messengers that are released from our body's endocrine glands and travel through the blood to elicit a specific response on another gland, organ, tissue, or cell in our body. They have the ability to bind to many different organs and cells, resulting in a different action at each binding site. For example, estrogen binds with receptors located on the uterus, breasts, brain, bladder, blood vessels, and bone, but will elicit a different response in each one. It stimulates the growth of uterine and breast tissue, keeps the bladder and urethra lining healthy, promotes blood-vessel dilation, and prevents bone loss. So, you can see that one hormone affects more than one organ in more than one way.

In addition to their ability to act on many different tissues, many hormones need to work together to elicit a specific action from a target tissue. For example, five hormones are needed to stimulate the release of your egg at ovulation: gonadotropin-releasing hormone, follicle-stimulating hormone, and luteinizing hormone, as well as estrogen and progesterone. All these hormones work together throughout the menstrual cycle to ensure ovulation. So, it's important to remember that many different hormones work together and influence each other's production and action. And when there is a hormonal imbalance, usually more than one hormone needs to be addressed.

Endocrine Glands and Their Hormones

The diagram below shows the different endocrine glands (glands that produce and release hormones).

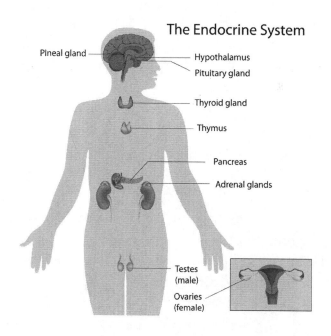

The Endocrine System

Pineal gland — Hypothalamus
Pituitary gland

Thyroid gland

Thymus

Pancreas

Adrenal glands

Testes (male)

Ovaries (female)

The pituitary gland, located in the brain and nicknamed the "master gland," controls the release of many different hormones. It secretes stimulating hormones that travel in the blood to other glands, promoting their release of hormones. Besides secreting these stimulating hormones, the pituitary gland also secretes growth hormone, prolactin, antidiuretic hormone, and oxytocin.

The pineal gland, like the pituitary gland, is found in the brain. It releases melatonin, the hormone responsible for regulating our daily circadian rhythm and sleep cycle.

The thyroid gland, found just behind the Adam's apple, governs our metabolism, weight, and energy by releasing thyroxine (T4) and triiodothyronine (T3).

The next set of important glands are the adrenal glands. These sit on top of the kidneys and release our stress hormones, as well as some sex hormones and a hormone to help us retain our water. Cortisol, dehydroepiandrosterone (DHEA), epinephrine, aldosterone, and some pregnenolone are all secreted by the adrenal glands to help our body cope with stress.

The pancreas is the gland that releases the hormone insulin to regulate our blood-sugar levels. It is the dysregulation of pancreatic hormones that plays a large role in insulin resistance and diabetes.

The sex organs (the testes and the ovaries) secrete the majority of our sex hormones: testosterone, estrogen, and progesterone respectively.

There are many different hormones, but I will cover only the hormones most commonly associated with hormonal imbalances I see in my practice: the thyroid hormones, cortisol, estrogens, progesterone, DHEA, and testosterone.

Thyroid Hormones

The thyroid hormones are responsible for regulating our metabolism, body temperature, and maintaining our weight and energy. The pituitary gland releases thyroid stimulating hormone (TSH) to stimulate the thyroid gland to secrete thyroxine (T4) and triiodothyronine (T3). T3 is considered the active hormone, which means it is the hormone that binds with other cells, tissues, and organs to kick our metabolism into gear, regulate our body temperature, and so on. Our bodies convert T4 into T3, not only in the thyroid gland, but also in the liver and gastrointestinal tract. So, if our liver and gastrointestinal tract are not functioning optimally because of nutritional deficiencies, toxins, or certain drugs, we may not be producing enough T3.

Low thyroid function (hypothyroidism) is one of the most common undiagnosed hormone imbalances I see in my practice. This is due in part to the inaccuracy of the so-called normal laboratory reference range for TSH. The reference range for TSH is currently set from 0.450–4.500 uIU/mL. This range is too wide, and anyone with a TSH greater than 2 uIU/mL can be experiencing hypothyroid symptoms. But when the majority of physicians see the TSH within this normal range, there is no further investigation of the thyroid gland. So, a large majority of people experiencing thyroid symptoms are not being treated.

People with low thyroid function can experience difficulty losing weight, headaches, low mood, fatigue, and lethargy, as well as chronic muscle soreness. As many of my patients explain, they just have no "oomph."

Estrogens

Estrogens have over 400 functions in our body. Many people think that estrogen is only a female hormone, but males also produce estrogen, just in smaller amounts. Estrogens are responsible for the female sex characteristics in women, such as breast development, the widened pelvis, and the distribution of fat around the hips and thighs. They also help regulate our blood pressure, promote arterial elasticity, and govern the female menstrual cycle, as well as maintain our energy, libido, mood, and memory. In addition, estrogen blocks bone loss, which is why postmenopausal women with decreased estrogen levels are at a higher risk of developing osteoporosis.

Types of Estrogen

There are actually three different types of estrogen: estrone, estradiol, and estriol. Estrone is the major source of estrogen after menopause. Estrone and its metabolites have been correlated with increased risk of breast and uterine cancer, so we don't want excess amounts of it. This is one of the problems with synthetic hormone replacement. The most common synthetic estrogen is 60-percent estrone, and since we already have enough of this during menopause, it is risky to provide more. Estradiol is the strongest estrogen and is at its highest levels in premenopausal women. It is the one estrogen that strongly promotes bone formation and prevents osteoporosis. The third estrogen is estriol. Estriol is nicknamed "the protective estrogen," as it doesn't appear to increase the growth of breast or uterine tissue. It is the weakest of all three of the estrogens and is found in high concentrations during pregnancy. Estriol and estradiol are the estrogens that are usually replaced during bioidentical hormone replacement therapy.

The female body starts producing higher levels of estrogen during puberty. During this time our pituitary gland releases follicle-stimulating hormone (FSH) and luteinizing hormone (LH), which then travel to the ovaries to stimulate the production and release of estrogen. This is when the female menstrual cycle starts to take form.

THE MENSTRUAL CYCLE EXPLAINED

The female reproductive cycle involves an interplay of hormones that normally results in cyclical changes in the ovaries and uterus. Each cycle takes approximately 28 days to complete and involves the development and release of an egg from the ovaries and the preparation of the uterus to receive a fertilized egg. If fertilization

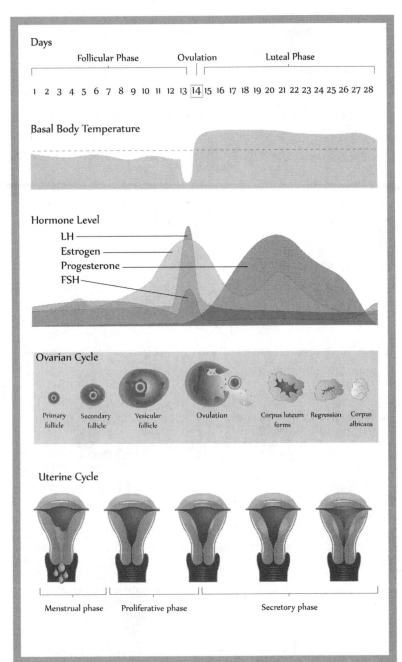

Days

Follicular Phase   Ovulation   Luteal Phase

1 2 3 4 5 6 7 8 9 10 11 12 13 14 15 16 17 18 19 20 21 22 23 24 25 26 27 28

Basal Body Temperature

Hormone Level
LH
Estrogen
Progesterone
FSH

Ovarian Cycle

Primary follicle   Secondary follicle   Vesicular follicle   Ovulation   Corpus luteum forms   Regression   Corpus albicans

Uterine Cycle

Menstrual phase   Proliferative phase   Secretory phase

doesn't occur, the endometrial (uterine) lining is lost through menstruation (day 1).

Follicular Phase

The first phase of the menstrual cycle is the follicular phase, beginning on the first day of menstrual bleeding. During this phase your pituitary gland starts releasing follicle-stimulating hormone (FSH) to stimulate the growth of the follicles contained in the ovaries. Each follicle contains an egg that is released during ovulation. The follicular phase usually lasts about 12 to 14 days and ends with an abrupt surge in luteinizing hormone to stimulate the release of the egg from the follicle.

Ovulatory Phase

Ovulation happens when the egg is released from the ovarian follicle. The egg then travels down the fallopian tubes, where it waits to be fertilized by the male sperm. This ovulatory phase lasts anywhere from 16 to 36 hours, but the egg can only be fertilized up to 12 hours after it has been released from the ovarian follicle.

Luteal Phase

The luteal phase begins right after ovulation. It lasts about 14 days, ending with menstruation. In this phase the follicle that released the egg forms a structure called the corpus luteum. The corpus luteum produces progesterone to help the body prepare for a possible pregnancy. Progesterone causes the cervical mucus to thicken to prevent bacteria and additional sperm from entering the uterus, while also increasing body temperature and helping to stimulate the thickening of the uterine lining along with estrogen.

If the egg is not fertilized, the corpus luteum degenerates, resulting in declining progesterone levels. This decline, accompanied by decreasing estrogen levels, signals the start of the menstrual period (menses). Menses occurs as the thickened uterine lining is slowly shed in order to prepare the uterus for the next menstrual cycle and possible fertilization.

If the egg is fertilized, the cells around the growing embryo produce human chorionic gonadotropin hormone, which will maintain the corpus luteum so it can continue its production of progesterone. Pregnancy tests are based on detecting increased levels of human chorionic gonadotropin.

Progesterone

Progesterone, like estrogen, has effects all over the body. It is responsible for maintaining pregnancy, protecting the heart and bones, regulating the menstrual cycle, increasing our mood, and decreasing anxiety, as well as promoting sleep. It also has potent anticancer characteristics in the breast and uterine tissues and is always prescribed along with estrogen replacement to block estrogen's proliferative action on these tissues. Progesterone plays a large role in a woman's mood and tranquility before her menstrual period and throughout pregnancy. It increases during the last half of the menstrual cycle in preparation for the implantation of a fertilized egg in the uterine wall and dramatically increases throughout pregnancy. If progesterone fails to increase to optimal levels during pregnancy, early miscarriages can result. Progesterone, like estrogen, decreases throughout menopause.

A NOTE ABOUT MENOPAUSE

Menopause usually occurs during your early fifties. However, some women can experience menopause as early as 35 years of age.

Menopause occurs when various hormones decline as a result of your ovaries starting to slow down. Estrogen and progesterone are primarily responsible for managing your menstrual cycle, so when those hormones decrease, your menstrual cycle is no longer stimulated, which results in the lessening of menstrual periods and eventually the complete absence of menses. Because your ovaries decrease production of estrogen and progesterone with menopause, it is up to your adrenal glands to take over. They will now have to produce extra estrogen and progesterone in addition to the testosterone, DHEA, and cortisol they are already producing. Because of this extra burden, the majority of hormones produced by the adrenal glands also decline with menopause. And it is this overall decline in hormones that results in the typical menopausal symptoms.

Testosterone

Many people think that testosterone is only a male hormone, but females also produce testosterone, just at lower concentrations: about 1/10 of the amount produced by males. Testosterone is the hormone that makes men "men" by promoting the male secondary sex characteristics, such as facial and body hair, narrow pelvis, and deepening of the voice, as well as increased muscle and bone strength. In both men and women, testosterone is often considered to be the sexy hormone as it is largely responsible for our sense of well-being, stamina, libido, and sexual desire. But testosterone doesn't only act as a sex hormone; it also protects the heart and blood vessels to reduce the risk of cardiovascular disease, maintains bone and muscle mass, decreases fat stores and obesity, and increases our sense of self-confidence.

In men testosterone is produced primarily by the testes, but in women the majority is produced and released by the adrenal glands, with a small amount being produced by the ovaries. In both men and women, testosterone declines dramatically with age. It has been shown that men between the ages of 50 and 70 have a lower testosterone level than the lowest level seen in men between 20 and 40 years old. And these men with the lower testosterone pass away sooner than men with higher testosterone levels.

DHEA

Dehydroepiandrosterone (DHEA), like testosterone, is a building hormone. It promotes energy, libido, and bone strength and helps our body heal from injury. It also acts to increase our mood and overall sense of well-being. In the past 10 years or so, it's been given credit as the "anti-aging hormone," because people who age well appear to have higher levels of DHEA than those who do not.

Lower DHEA levels are associated with the risk of developing type II diabetes, cardiovascular disorders, and inflammatory conditions such as arthritis, as well as some cancers. A special function of DHEA comes from its ability to convert into estrogen and testosterone when needed and to oppose the effects of excess cortisol and stress.

DHEA is synthesized primarily in the adrenal glands, with a small amount produced in the brain. By the age of 70, DHEA levels decline as much as 90 percent, resulting in some of the symptoms and conditions associated with aging.

Cortisol

Cortisol is considered our stress hormone. It is produced by the adrenal glands and is responsible for the flight-or-fight response; we see a bear, we get scared, and our cortisol (along with other stress hormones) kicks in to prepare our body for the stress of either fighting the bear or running from it. Some of these typical acute stress responses include pupil dilation, increased blood-sugar levels, the temporary shutdown of our digestive and immune systems, and the rerouting of blood away from our internal organs toward our brain and skeletal muscles.

Our bodies are programmed to release cortisol in times of stress. The problem is that stress should be only temporary; for example, we see the bear and we decide to run from it. After we get away from the bear and feel safe again, the stress response dissipates and our cortisol levels return to normal. However, stress is more chronic these days. Stressful jobs, meeting deadlines, taking care of our families, working long hours, and eating a nutrient-deficient diet all stimulate the stress response. As a result, our adrenal glands are forced to release cortisol at higher levels for a longer time than normal. Over time our adrenal glands become tired, resulting in burnout and symptoms of adrenal fatigue. So, it's important to find ways to monitor and cope effectively with our stress.

In addition to cortisol's antistress actions, it also decreases inflammation and allergies and improves concentration, energy and mood.

Now that we have discussed what hormones are and what they do for you, let's move on to diagnosing your specific hormonal imbalances so you can pinpoint the best treatment program for your needs.

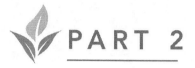

PART 2

Hormone Diagnosis: Questionnaire, Symptoms, and Lab Testing

CHAPTER 3

Happy Hormones Questionnaire

I N E A C H of the following tables, rate the severity of your symptoms:

0 = none
1 = mild
2 = moderate
3 = severe

After you have rated the severity of your symptoms, total the score at the bottom of each test and compare with the given assessment scores.

If your results indicate a possible deficiency or probable deficiency, please refer to Part 3 to learn more about your treatment options for each hormone imbalance.

ESTROGEN DEFICIENCY	
	Score
Hot flashes and night sweats	
Poor memory and forgetfulness	
Dribbling of urine upon coughing or sneezing	
Dry and irritated eyes	
Thin facial wrinkles around eyes and lips	
Low mood and/or depression	
Decreased breast firmness	
Low libido	
Irregular menstrual cycles	
Light menstrual flow	
Painful intercourse due to vaginal dryness	
Easily broken bones	
Osteopenia or osteoporosis	
Total:	

Assessment:

12 or less = sufficient levels

Between 13 and 23 = possible deficiency

More than 23 = probable deficiency

ESTROGEN EXCESS	Score
Heavy menstrual bleeding	
Weight gain around the hips and thighs	
Uterine fibroids	
Irritability and low mood	
Painful menstrual cramps	
Breast swelling and tenderness	
Anxiety	
Irritable and more emotional before menstrual period	
Total:	

Assessment:

    8 or less = balanced levels

    Between 9 and 16 = possible excess

    More than 16 = probable excess

PROGESTERONE DEFICIENCY	Score
Difficulty sleeping	
Anxiety and nervousness	
Easily irritated and agitated	
Low mood and/or depression	
Tender, swollen breasts before menstrual period	
Irritable and more emotional before menstrual period	
Heavy menstrual periods	
Painful menstrual cramps	
Abdominal bloating before menstrual period	
Uterine fibroids and/or ovarian cysts	
Infertility	
History of miscarriages	
Total:	

Assessment:

Postmenopausal women:
    4 or less = sufficient levels
    Between 5 and 8 = possible deficiency
    More than 8 = probable deficiency

Premenopausal women and women taking hormone replacement therapy:
    12 or less = sufficient levels
    Between 13 and 23 = possible deficiency
    More than 23 = probable deficiency

TESTOSTERONE DEFICIENCY Men and women:	Score
Loss of muscle tone	
Increased abdominal fat	
Tiredness	
Decreased libido	
Hot flashes and/or night sweats	
Lower self-esteem and lack of confidence	
Men only:	
Loss of breast (pectoral) muscle tone	
Decreased endurance during exercise	
Decreased sexual performance	
Total:	

Assessment:

Women:

    6 or less = sufficient levels

    Between 7 and 11 = possible deficiency

    More than 12 = probable deficiency

Men:

    9 or less = sufficient levels

    Between 10 and 20 = possible deficiency

    More than 20 = probable deficiency

DHEA (DEHYDROEPIANDROSTERONE) DEFICIENCY	Score
Loss of muscle tone	
Increased abdominal fat	
Loss of body hair (underarms and pubic hair)	
Decreased concentration	
Lack of focus	
Decreased tolerance to noise	
Low libido	
Total:	

Assessment:
    7 or less = sufficient levels
    Between 8 and 14 = possible deficiency
    More than 14 = probable deficiency

TESTOSTERONE AND DHEA EXCESS	
	Score
Increased facial hair	
Menstrual cycle longer than 35 days	
Absence of menstrual period	
Greasy skin and hair	
Acne	
Blood-sugar dysregulation (high or low)	
Infertility	
Irritability and aggression	
Polycystic ovarian syndrome	
Total:	

Assessment:
    9 or less = balanced levels
    Between 10 and 18 = possible excess
    More than 18 = probable excess

CORTISOL DEFICIENCY	
	Score
Difficulty concentrating and inability to focus	
Crying bouts for no particular reason	
Increased irritability and agitation to things that were never a bother in the past	
Fatigue, worse in the afternoon	
Difficulty coping with stress	
Decreased tolerance to noise	
Low blood pressure	
Digestion complaints (gas, bloating, abdominal cramps/pain)	
Salt and sugar cravings	
Increased frequency of colds and flu	
Cravings for coffee and other stimulants	
Environmental and/or food allergies	
Eczema, psoriasis, hives, and other skin rashes	
Fatigue during or after exercise	
Total:	

Assessment:

    14 or less = sufficient levels

    Between 15 and 26 = possible deficiency

    More than 26 = probable deficiency

CORTISOL EXCESS	Score
Stressed out	
Difficulty sleeping	
Abdominal weight gain	
Wired feeling	
Feeling of running on adrenaline	
Easily irritated	
Thinning skin or itchy, irritated skin	
Increased frequency of colds and flu	
High blood pressure	
Irregular menstrual cycles	
Unexplained infertility	
Total:	

Assessment:

11 or more = elevated cortisol levels, indicating active stress

THYROID DEFICIENCY	Score
Intolerance to cold	
Cold hands and feet	
Difficulty getting up in the morning	
Constant fatigue	
Recurrent headaches	
Easy weight gain	
Dry skin	
Dry and brittle hair and nails	
Constipation, not having regular daily bowel movements	
Loss of outer one-third of eyebrows	
Low mood or depression	
Taking antidepressants that don't seem to make a difference with mood	
Family history of thyroid problems	
Total:	

Assessment:

    12 or less = sufficient levels

    Between 13 and 23 = possible deficiency

    More than 23 = probable deficiency

CHAPTER 4

Symptoms of Hormonal Imbalances

W HEN LOOKING at hormonal imbalances, there is often more than one imbalance occurring at a time. Hormones all influence each other, and because of this we often see a combination of imbalances.

The diagram on the following page shows the complexity of hormone interaction. You can see that different hormones are needed for the production of others, so if there is a deficiency or excess in one hormone, there will most likely be an imbalance of the other hormones down that same path. Because of this chain reaction, it is necessary to look at more than just one hormone in order to gain a thorough understanding of what is happening with your overall balance. Without this big-picture perspective, you will be unable to effectively assess and treat your hormonal imbalances.

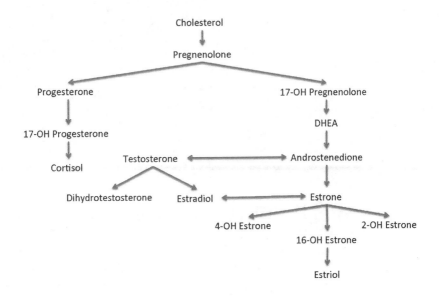

Cortisol

Cortisol is the body's major defense against stress, both physical and emotional. Physical stress can occur from injuries, infections, excessive exercise, malnutrition, changes in body temperature, inflammation, and more. Emotional stress arises from daily pressures, loss of loved ones, emotional traumas, and other factors affecting our mental state. Without cortisol we would be unable to cope with these stressors. It is the one hormone we need to survive.

Cortisol Excess

Cortisol imbalance begins with stress. Our bodies produce and secrete higher levels of cortisol in response to stress to help us cope with whatever the stressor may be. However, this stress is designed to be a short-term process, not for the days, months, and years that chronic stress is today.

Symptoms of excess cortisol are often associated with the typical stress symptoms: anxiety, irritability, sleep disturbance, and a wired feeling. If the stress goes on long enough, you can experience loss of muscle and bone mass as cortisol breaks down your proteins, along with thinning skin and an increased susceptibility to illness because cortisol suppresses the immune system.

SYMPTOMS OF HIGH CORTISOL	
Anxiety	Thinning skin
Insomnia	Insulin resistance
Stressed-out feeling	Irritability
Abdominal weight gain	High blood pressure
Loss of muscle and bone mass	Increased frequency of colds and flu

I often see high cortisol levels in clients with stressful jobs, as well as in new moms and university and graduate-school students.

If this stress continues, our adrenal glands can have a hard time keeping up. They may be unable to produce enough cortisol to meet our daily demands, resulting in lower cortisol levels and eventually adrenal fatigue.

Adrenal Fatigue Progression

Adrenal fatigue is essentially the collection of signs and symptoms resulting from low cortisol levels. Your cortisol levels normally increase with stress, and then decrease back to normal levels within a period of a few hours. But with today's chronic stress, our cortisol levels remain higher than normal to cope with these stress demands (called the resistance phase). If this stress continues for a long period of time, our adrenal glands can begin to have a hard time keeping up with the cortisol demands. Cortisol levels then begin to decline, resulting in the typical adrenal fatigue symptoms (see diagram below).

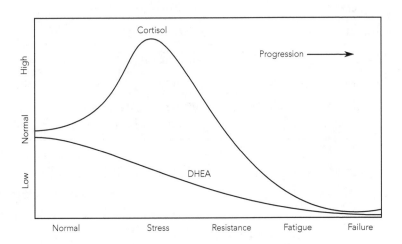

The time frame within the different phases of adrenal fatigue varies greatly between individuals. Some people manage their high cortisol levels for their entire life, whereas other people progress quite quickly from the resistance phase into adrenal fatigue. Sometimes people can coast along in the resistance phase until an acute stress occurs, such as the loss of a loved one. This stress can push them rapidly into adrenal fatigue. I often hear clients say, "since this particular event, I haven't been the same," or, "since this event, I've had no energy, problems dealing with stress, and am constantly sick."

Cortisol Deficiency

Cortisol deficiency (also known as adrenal fatigue) is something I am seeing more and more in my practice. I often see this in people who lead busy lives and are under a lot of stress. For example, university students, working mothers, people in high-stakes jobs, and people with a history of abuse and family/relationship difficulties or losses. Adrenal fatigue is one of the most common and underdiagnosed hormone imbalances. The reason why cortisol deficiency is not readily diagnosed is because it's not looked for in conventional medicine, and the blood tests focus on adrenal *failure*, not fatigue.

SYMPTOMS OF LOW CORTISOL	
Anxiety	Difficulty concentrating
Inability to cope with stress	Low blood pressure
Easily irritated	Asthma
Fatigue	Increased frequency of colds and flu
Worsened allergies (environmental and food)	Eczema, psoriasis, and other skin rashes
Salt and sugar cravings	

One thing to note is the adrenal glands' role after menopause. These glands are the primary source of sex hormones after menopause, so if they are tired and struggling to produce enough cortisol for our daily needs, our estrogen, progesterone, DHEA, and testosterone levels will decrease faster than they would with healthy, functioning adrenal glands. This can result in the worsening of menopause symptoms.

Testosterone

Many people think of testosterone as just a male hormone, but it's also an important female hormone. Men have about 10 times the amount of testosterone than women, and it's these higher levels that are responsible for the male secondary sex characteristics. Testosterone is a building hormone, so it plays a large role in maintaining our muscle and bone mass and provides us with an overall sense of confidence, energy, and well-being.

Testosterone Deficiency

Testosterone levels start declining in our mid-twenties but symptoms usually do not arise until menopause and andropause (the state resulting from declining levels of testosterone in men).

SYMPTOMS OF LOW TESTOSTERONE	
Decreased libido	Night sweats
Fatigue	Hot flashes
Increased abdominal fat	Aches and pains
Loss of bone and muscle mass	Facial wrinkles
Decreased sexual performance in men	Lack of self-confidence

Testosterone Excess

I usually see high testosterone levels only in someone taking too high a dose of exogenous testosterone or in women with polycystic ovarian syndrome (PCOS). High testosterone levels can lead to symptoms of aggression, increased facial hair, and acne. PCOS is a common cause of amenorrhea (absence of menstrual period) and infertility in women, so if you are experiencing these symptoms, do have your testosterone levels checked and PCOS ruled out.

SYMPTOMS OF HIGH TESTOSTERONE	
Excessive facial hair (women)	Irritability and/or aggression
Ovarian cysts (women)	Oily skin and hair
Acne	Infertility (women)

DHEA

Dehydroepiandrosterone (DHEA), like testosterone, is a building hormone. However, it is produced and released by the adrenal glands, so it is important to note that symptoms of excess or low DHEA can often mimic both testosterone and cortisol imbalances.

DHEA Deficiency

DHEA levels start declining in our early thirties, but like testosterone, symptoms usually do not appear until later. However, if there is chronic stress, DHEA levels can decline quicker, resulting in an earlier onset of symptoms.

SYMPTOMS OF LOW DHEA	
Loss of muscle tone	Difficulty concentrating
Increased abdominal fat	Decreased libido
Loss of body hair (pubic and underarms)	Decreased tolerance to noise

DHEA *Excess*

Excess DHEA is usually seen only in someone with adrenal disease, acute stress, polycystic ovarian syndrome (PCOS), or someone taking excessive amounts of DHEA supplements. Over the past few years, I have been seeing more and more women with PCOS showing high DHEA levels.

SYMPTOMS OF HIGH DHEA	
Oily skin and acne	Sugar cravings
Excessive facial hair (women)	Mood changes

Estrogen

Estrogen, like testosterone, is important for both men and women, only in the reverse amounts: women have more, men have less. Estrogens are responsible for the secondary sex characteristics in women, such as breast development, widening of the pelvis, and the distribution of fat around the hips and the thighs. It has many effects on different tissues, including the brain, breasts, thyroid, and bone. Estrogen actually blocks bone loss, which is why postmenopausal women with decreased estrogen levels are at a higher risk of developing osteoporosis.

As mentioned earlier, there are three different types of estrogen: estrone, estradiol, and estriol. For a quick review of these estrogens, please refer back to Chapter 2: "What Are Hormones and Why Are They Important?"

Estrogen Deficiency

Estrogen deficiency is most often seen in postmenopausal women. Throughout menopause the ovaries slowly decrease their estrogen production, and it is up to our adrenal glands to take over. However, usually by this point in our lives, our adrenal glands are tired and are having a hard enough time just producing enough cortisol. As a result, our estrogen levels, which are already naturally declining, can decline even quicker. Symptoms of this estrogen deficiency are the typical menopause symptoms.

SYMPTOMS OF LOW ESTROGEN	
Hot flashes and night sweats	Dry skin
Dribbling of urine upon coughing or sneezing	Dry, irritated eyes
Wrinkles around eyes and lips	Bone loss, osteoporosis
Low mood and depression	Foggy thinking
Vaginal dryness	Memory lapses
Irregular menstrual cycles	Hair loss

Estrogen Excess

Estrogen excess is a condition that I am seeing more and more in my practice. Our environment is filled with xenoestrogens, chemicals that mimic estrogen in our body. These xenoestrogens are found in many different plastics, cleaning supplies, cosmetics, water, and meat and dairy products. Xenoestrogens build up in our bodies, causing abnormally high levels of estrogen and estrogen-excess symptoms. Estrogen excess usually goes hand in hand with progesterone deficiency, so these two conditions have similar PMS-type symptoms.

SYMPTOMS OF HIGH ESTROGEN	
Difficulty sleeping	Anxiety and nervousness
Easily irritated and agitated	Low mood or depression
Heavy menstrual periods	Menstrual cramps
Fibrocystic breasts	Uterine fibroids
Tender, swollen breasts before menstrual period	Irritable and more emotional before menstrual period

Progesterone

Progesterone, like estrogen, has receptors all over the body. Until about 30 years ago, a woman who had a complete hysterectomy (which is the removal of the ovaries and uterus) was given only estrogen and not progesterone because doctors at the time thought that progesterone influenced only the uterus. But they were so wrong. Progesterone has many different functions throughout the body; it not only maintains pregnancy and helps regulate the menstrual cycle, but it also acts as a natural antidepressant, protects the breasts from excess estrogen, and is a cardiovascular protectant. It is an important hormone to keep at optimal levels.

Progesterone Deficiency

Throughout menopause progesterone levels slowly decline, leading to many different symptoms. However, I have noticed more and more premenopausal women also presenting with progesterone deficiencies, such as PMS and/or difficulty conceiving. Low progesterone levels during pregnancy have been associated with an increased risk of first trimester miscarriages, so it is important to ensure you have adequate levels during pregnancy.

SYMPTOMS OF LOW PROGESTERONE	
Difficulty sleeping	Anxiety and nervousness
Easily irritated and agitated	Low mood or depression
Heavy menstrual periods	Menstrual cramps
History of miscarriages	Uterine fibroids
Tender, swollen breasts before menstrual period	Irritable and more emotional before menstrual period

Progesterone Excess

Progesterone excess is not very common. I usually see it only in women taking too high a dose of bioidentical or synthetic progesterone.

SYMPTOMS OF HIGH PROGESTERONE	
Drowsiness and depression	Nausea
Increased acne and facial hair	Breast swelling

Thyroid Hormones

The thyroid hormones are important for maintaining our metabolism, body temperature, and energy levels. If there is an imbalance with these hormones, you can experience changes in weight, energy, appetite, and body temperature.

Thyroid Deficiency

Thyroid deficiency is called hypothyroidism. Like adrenal fatigue, it is currently one of the most underdiagnosed conditions. The problem is that hypothyroidism isn't being readily diagnosed; the normal reference range for thyroid hormones is much too wide, so many people with low thyroid symptoms are told they have normal results and are given no further testing or treatment. If you suspect hypothyroidism but your doctor tells you that your results are normal, I highly suggest you go for a second opinion to a health professional familiar with thyroid diagnosis and treatment.

Thyroid hormone production and metabolism is quite complex and is often influenced by many different factors. Nutritional deficiencies, stress, autoimmunity, digestive disturbances, and fluctuation of your other hormones can all influence your thyroid function.

SYMPTOMS OF LOW THYROID	
Fatigue and low mood	Constipation
Difficulty getting up in the morning	Headaches and migraines
Difficultly losing weight	Cold hands and feet
Menstrual cramps	Sensitivity to cold
Dry skin and hair	Hair loss
Loss of lateral one-third of eyebrows	

Thyroid Excess

An excess of thyroid hormones is called hyperthyroidism. It is usually caused by an autoimmune response toward the thyroid gland. Hyperthyroidism is readily diagnosed in comparison to hypothyroidism and usually does not fall through the cracks of the medical system.

SYMPTOMS OF HIGH THYROID	
Increased weight loss	Frequent bowel movements
Increased appetite	Rapid heartbeat
Anxiety, nervousness	Frequent sweating
Menstrual cramps	Muscle weakness
Tremors	

CHAPTER 5

Recommended Laboratory Testing

L ABORATORY TESTING is used as a confirmation in the diagnoses of various hormonal imbalances. There are many different types of lab tests, including blood, urine, and saliva. All three of these are useful when testing hormone levels.

Blood Tests

Below is a list of the hormones I typically test in the blood:

Female Blood Profile
    Complete blood count
    Chemistry panel
    Lipid panel
    FSH, LH

TSH, free T4, free T3
Estradiol, estrone and estriol
Progesterone
Total and free testosterone
Dihydrotestosterone (DHT)
Sex hormone-binding globulin (SHBG)
Vitamin D3
Vitamin B12
Ferritin
DHEAs
C-reactive protein

Male Blood Profile
Complete blood count
Chemistry panel
Lipid panel
Prostate specific antigen (PSA), percentage free PSA
TSH, free T4, free T3
Estradiol
Progesterone
Total and free testosterone
Dihydrotestosterone (DHT)
Sex hormone-binding globulin (SHBG)
Vitamin D3
Vitamin B12
DHEAs
C-reactive protein

Follicle-stimulating hormone (FSH) and luteinizing hormone (LH) are tested to help determine if a woman is ovulating, in menopause, or if PCOS is a concern. These hormones normally increase in postmenopausal women because they are trying to signal your ovaries to produce more estrogen and progesterone.

Estradiol, estrone, progesterone, testosterone, and DHEA are tested to confirm deficiencies or excesses of these hormones, and also to monitor treatment and dosages if using bioidentical hormones. TSH, free T4, and free T3 are measured to assess if there is a thyroid hormone deficiency or excess. Vitamin B12, vitamin D3, and iron are very common deficiencies, so these are always part of my routine testing. In order to evaluate iron stores, I always test ferritin, as it is a more accurate determinant of iron status. Iron deficiency is very common in premenopausal women due to the monthly menstrual cycles.

C-reactive protein (CRP) is a marker of inflammation that is tested to help evaluate the risk of future heart disease and inflammatory conditions.

The complete blood count (CBC), chemistry panel, and lipid panel are used to evaluate your blood cells, electrolytes, and cholesterol levels. These are all baseline tests that are routinely checked with your annual physical exam.

There are some additional tests for men, one of which is called prostate-specific antigen (PSA). This test is used to evaluate inflammation and cancer of the prostate gland, as well as to help determine the aggressiveness of the cancer and monitor prostate cancer treatment progress. Every man above the age of 30 should have his PSA levels monitored yearly.

Below I have included my optimal values for a few of the hormones tested in the blood. These values differ from the set normal reference ranges given by the laboratory, as I feel some of the set ranges are too wide.

Hormone	Female	Male
TSH	0.8–2 mIU/L	0.8–2 mIU/L
Free T4	Upper third of reference range	Upper third of reference range
Free T3	Upper third of reference range	Upper third of reference range
Total testosterone	50–80 ng/dl	700–1,000 ng/dl
Free testosterone	1.0–2.3 pg/ml	18–28 pg/dl
DHEAs	150–300 ug/dl	400–600 ug/dl
Progesterone (postmeno-pausal)	2–8 pg/ml	
Progesterone (premenopausal women on day 21 of menstrual cycle)	15–23 ng/ml	
Estradiol (post-menopausal)	80–200 pg/ml	
Estradiol (pre-menopausal)	80–400 pg/ml	

Salivary Tests

Saliva samples are used in the evaluation of cortisol levels. Free cortisol easily passes into tissues, making saliva samples an accurate measure of the actual amounts of cortisol affecting our tissues and glands. I also prefer salivary cortisol testing because blood cortisol levels can be falsely elevated. Having your blood drawn is a stressful situation, and when we are stressed, our body releases cortisol, resulting in higher serum concentrations. In these cases, a cortisol deficiency may be hidden because the acute stress of the blood draw increases blood cortisol levels, resulting in your cortisol levels appearing normal when they may actually be low.

Cortisol saliva samples are collected at four different times over the course of one day. Cortisol has a natural daily rhythm, with levels increasing early in the morning and slowly decreasing through the afternoon and evening. By taking cortisol at four separate times, we get a more accurate assessment.

Urinary Tests

Urine is incredibly useful for testing hormone metabolites and assessing estradiol, estrone, estriol, cortisol, and testosterone levels.

Urinary Metabolite Testing
  2-hydroxyestrone
  16a-hydroxyestrone
  5a-androstanediol
  5b-androstanediol

Sometimes estrogen and testosterone are metabolized into unwanted and potentially harmful by-products. Because of this, it is important to measure these metabolites to ensure optimal metabolism and conversion of your hormones, particularly when using bioidentical hormones.

I recommend discussing the tests most appropriate for you with your health-care provider. Some tests may be omitted, while others may need to be added. When you receive the results, you can then review them together with your health-care provider to develop a treatment program suitable for your specific imbalances. If your doctor is not on board with testing your hormones, I have included a list of labs offering home testing in the Appendix.

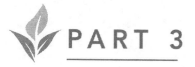

PART 3

Happy Hormones
Treatment Program

CHAPTER 6

Nutrition for Happy Hormones

Why Nutrition Is Important

When it comes to balancing hormones, the first place to start is with a healthy eating program. Many foods benefit our natural production and balance of hormones, whereas other foods can decrease production of beneficial hormones, increase production of hormone disruptors, and decrease our detoxification pathways.

Quite often you can restore your hormone health just by adapting a healthy eating program. We are what we eat, so if you eat a healthy, balanced diet, your body will also come into balance. You can be well on your way to balanced hormones and a healthier body and mind simply by following these guidelines.

By following this general nutrition program, you will notice increased energy, better sleep, weight loss (if not already at your optimal weight), and less digestive disturbance. Try not to think of this program as a diet. It is merely a set of guidelines to help you have a more nutrient-rich diet so your body can function at its full capacity. Some people find it helpful to have a "free" day, as this will decrease the urge of wanting what you can't have. Once a week go out and enjoy dinner with friends or have that food you've been thinking about all week.

After following this program for a few weeks, you will notice a significant decrease in your food cravings. Once our bodies get accustomed to eating healthy whole foods, the desire and taste for sweets and more processed foods decreases. You won't feel that same satisfaction you did before when you eat them. So, try your best to stick to the guidelines for the first few weeks to give your body time to get used to the healthier, natural foods and develop its "do not eat" signal for junk food.

Foods to Eat Freely

The foods that must comprise the majority of your diet are foods that we have eaten for thousands of years that are found naturally in the environment and have not been altered by today's manufacturing processes. These foods are organic vegetables, fruits, lean meats, eggs, seeds, herbs, spices, and fish.

Organic Vegetables

Vegetables are high in many vitamins, minerals, antioxidants, and fiber. All of these are necessary to maintain hormonal balance and overall health in general. We have been eating vegetables since the very beginning, so our bodies are quite efficient at digesting and utilizing the nutrients obtained from them.

It is important to buy organic vegetables to avoid exposure to the pesticides and herbicides that are so commonly sprayed on them. These chemicals have many health-related risks.

The vegetables to focus on include:

Brassica vegetables
- Broccoli
- Brussels sprouts
- Cabbage
- Cauliflower
- Collard greens
- Turnips

Allium vegetables
- Chives
- Garlic
- Leeks
- Onion
- Shallots

Leafy greens
- Beet greens
- Cilantro
- Collard greens
- Dark lettuce
- Kale
- Mustard greens
- Parsley
- Spinach

Others
- Asparagus
- Beets
- Carrots
- Celery
- Cucumber
- Radishes
- Red and
  yellow peppers
- Squash
- Tomatoes
- Zucchini

Organic Fruit

Like vegetables, fruit contains vitamins, minerals, antioxidants, and fiber. We can easily digest, absorb, and utilize the nutrients found in fruit. However, some fruits are also high in sugar and should be eaten only occasionally. These fruits include pineapple, mango, papaya, and other tropical fruits It is important to buy organic fruit to avoid exposure to the pesticides and herbicides that are so commonly sprayed on the fruit trees. These chemicals have many health-related risks.

The fruits to incorporate into your program include:
- All berries
- Apples
- Apricots
- Cherries
- Kiwis
- Lemons
- Limes
- Nectarines
- Pears
- Plums

Organic Lean Meats and Eggs

It's important to ensure adequate protein intake. Protein is needed to maintain muscle and bone mass, energy, detoxification, and hormone production. However, you must be cautious with meat as many types of meat contain traces of antibiotics, hormones, and nitrates, all of which disrupt hormone balance and the immune system.

Rule of thumb: Eat organic, grass-fed, hormone-free, and antibiotic-free meat in moderation.

The lean animal protein you should incorporate into your program includes:

- Organic bison
- Organic chicken and turkey
- Organic eggs
- Wild game

Seeds and Healthy Oils

Seeds and oils, such as pumpkin seeds, chia seeds, olive oil, coconut oil, and flaxseed oil, contain healthy fats called omega-3 fatty acids. These omega-3 fatty acids are natural anti-inflammatories, support our immune system, and play a critical role in hormone production. Seeds also contain vitamins and minerals, such as zinc, selenium, and B vitamins, which are vital for optimal hormonal balance.

The healthy fats found in seeds and oils are necessary to build our cell membranes, allow for nerve transmission, protect our organs, and support the production of so many different hormones. There are some fats, however, that we do not need in our diet. These are the fats that are superheated, overcooked, or burnt. High temperatures change the structure of the fat, making it unhealthy for us, so avoid fats and oils heated at high temperatures.

Rule of thumb: Include healthy, unheated fats, oils, and seeds in your diet.

Seeds and oils you can incorporate into your program include:

Oils
- Coconut oil
- Flaxseed oil
- Olive oil

Seeds
- Chia seeds
- Flaxseeds
- Hemp seeds
- Pumpkin seeds
- Sesame seeds
- Sunflower seeds

Seafood

Fish contains the same healthy fatty acids as oils and seeds. However, fish is prone to mercury contamination, so it is important to eat only fish containing the lowest mercury levels. It is beneficial to focus on small, fatty fish from cold bodies of water, as they have higher amounts of omega-3 fatty acids and lower amounts of mercury.

Rule of thumb: Include small, cold-water fish into your diet and avoid larger fish, like tuna or swordfish.

Fish to incorporate into your program include:

- Anchovies
- Arctic cod
- Catfish
- Mackerel
- Perch
- Plaice
- Pollock
- Salmon
- Sardines
- Sole
- Tilapia
- Trout (freshwater)
- Whitefish

Herbs and Spices

Herbs and spices have been used for thousands of years to treat all kinds of illnesses and afflictions. Some have antibacterial or anti-inflammatory properties, while others work to increase circulation, promote healthy digestion, or elevate mood. Plus they add flavor and color to your meals. Experiment with different herbs and spices to find out which ones you enjoy the most.

Herbs and spices to incorporate into your program include:

- Basil
- Black pepper
- Cardamom
- Cayenne pepper
- Celery seed
- Cinnamon
- Cloves
- Coriander
- Cumin
- Dill
- Fennel
- Garlic
- Ginger
- Mustard seeds

- Nutmeg
- Oregano
- Rosemary
- Sage

- Thyme
- Turmeric
- Vanilla bean

Water and Unsweetened, Caffeine-Free Herbal Tea

Be sure to drink at least two liters of water or herbal tea per day. If your water source is chlorinated or fluorinated, purchase a highly rated water filter to filter out those contaminants. There are many different kinds of filters: some attach to your faucet, while others are mounted underneath the sink or sit on the countertop.

Bottled water does not count as filtered water. Bottled water is surrounded by plastic, which eventually leaches harmful chemicals into the water. These plastic chemicals are incredible hormone disruptors and need to be completely avoided.

Coffee and tea plants are heavily sprayed with pesticides, so try to use organic tea as much as possible.

Rule of thumb: Drink filtered water, not from a plastic water bottle, and use this filtered water to make caffeine-free, organic herbal teas.

Foods to Eat in Moderation

Red Meats

Red meat should be eaten in moderation, as it has been linked to an increased risk of heart disease. Red meat contains saturated fats and high amounts of arachidonic acid, a compound that leads to inflammation in the body. Inflammation is a precursor to many illnesses, including cardiovascular disease and cancer.

Furthermore, red meat is often contaminated with colorings, antibiotics, and hormones, making it a somewhat processed food. So when you do have red meat, ensure it is organic, grass-fed, antibiotic-free, and hormone-free.

Rule of thumb: Red meats should be eaten only occasionally and must be organic, grass-fed, antibiotic-free, and hormone-free.

Nuts and Legumes

Nuts are full of healthy oils, and legumes (such as beans and peas) are great sources of protein. The downside to these is that they are difficult for us to digest. They contain compounds that inhibit the enzymes necessary for their digestion and metabolism. However, if you sprout or cook your nuts and beans, these enzymes are deactivated, making them much easier for your body to digest.

One nut to avoid completely is the peanut. Peanuts are more prone to fungal contamination, which, when eaten, can contribute to the growth of candida (yeast-like fungi) in the intestines. Candida overgrowth can be the cause of gas, bloating, fatigue, and even weight gain. Peanuts, like red meat, also contain arachidonic acid and are great at activating our immune system, triggering an allergic response.

Rule of thumb: Sprout or cook your legumes before eating; limit to three times per week.

Whole Grains

Whole grains contain many essential vitamins and minerals, but like legumes and nuts, they are difficult for us to digest. Be sure to cook your grains thoroughly before eating and keep the portion to no more than ¼ cup cooked with each meal.

Rule of thumb: Cook your grains.

Some grains to incorporate into your nutrition program include:

- Amaranth
- Brown rice
- Millet
- Quinoa

Foods to Avoid

Wheat and Gluten

About 85 percent of people I see in my practice have wheat and gluten sensitivities. This sensitivity results in symptoms of Crohn's disease, ulcerative colitis, irritable bowel syndrome (IBS), low mood, weight gain, and low energy. I have seen the elimination of gluten and wheat dramatically improve health.

Foods containing wheat and gluten that must be avoided include:

- Bread
- Candy
- Meat replacements
- Packaged foods
- Pasta
- Pastries and baked goods

Foods Containing Yeast

Any food containing yeast will contribute to the overgrowth of candida in the intestines, which can then spread to other areas, such as the skin, vagina, etc.

Symptoms of candida overgrowth include constipation, abdominal bloating, gas, fungal skin infections, skin rashes, weight gain, and fatigue. If you have any of these symptoms, completely avoid foods containing sugar and yeast.

The foods containing yeast that must be avoided are:

- Alcohol
- Breads
- Cheese
- Pastries and baked goods

Coffee and Black Tea

Both coffee and black teas are diuretics, which lead to dehydration by increasing urine output. This dehydration is often the culprit in difficult digestion, constipation, headaches, and dry, wrinkly skin.

Caffeine also stimulates the stress response. Over time this stress response can contribute to a hormonal imbalance by overworking the adrenal glands. The adrenal glands are responsible for our cortisol and DHEA production, as well as some testosterone, progesterone, and estrogen production in postmenopausal women. They are crucial for our overall hormonal balance and often need extra support.

Substitutions: You can substitute coffee and black tea with water and herbal, caffeine-free tea.

Alcohol

Alcohol not only contributes to candida overgrowth, but it also burdens your liver. The liver is the main organ responsible for detoxification of our hormones and waste products. If it is busy dealing with the detoxification of alcohol, it won't have time to rid our body of these excess hormones or waste products.

Condiments and Sauces

Condiments are often loaded with salt, sugar, colorings, preservatives, and flavorings. There is very little natural about them. Avoid these as much as possible, and when you do have them, ensure it is only in small amounts.

Substitutions: Experiment at home by making your own salad dressings (olive oil, balsamic vinegar, and lemon juice), sauces (homemade hummus, pesto, salsa, and guacamole), and marinades; See the "Happy Hormones Recipe Collection" in the Appendix for more ideas.

Sugar and Foods Containing Sugar

Candida love sugar and will rapidly grow in its presence. Sugar also significantly decreases our immune system, rendering it susceptible to various bacterial and viral infections and cancer. A diet high in sugar also contributes to low energy and an increased risk of diabetes.

High-fructose corn syrup must be avoided at all costs. This substance has been linked with excess weight gain and obesity, as well as diabetes and heart disease. Check all of your condiments for high-fructose corn syrup and, if it contains it, throw it out.

Sugar sources to be aware of include:

- Galactose
- High-fructose corn syrup
- Honey
- Lactose
- Maltose
- Maple syrup
- Molasses
- Products containing sugar
- Sorbitol
- Sucrose

Dairy Products

We are not designed to digest dairy products. No other animal drinks milk past infancy, and we shouldn't either. The enzymes needed to digest breast milk decrease throughout childhood, so as adults, we have an incredibly hard time digesting it.

Because of this lack of enzymes, the dairy products we eat can end up sitting in our intestines for up to three days before they're fully digested. This results in an overgrowth of candida and an increase in fermentation. This process creates digestive difficulty with gas and bloating, as well as a state of toxicity.

The dairy industry has us believing that dairy products are the only source of calcium, but this is absolutely untrue. You can find calcium in higher levels than many dairy products in the following foods:

Foods containing calcium include:

- Almonds
- Beans
- Blackstrap molasses
- Broccoli
- Collard greens
- Dark, leafy greens
- Figs
- Spinach
- Tempeh
- Tofu

Packaged and Processed Foods

Canned, bottled, boxed, and other packaged and processed foods usually contain refined sugar products, preservatives, and colorings, as well as other harmful hidden ingredients. These need to be completely avoided.

Breads, Pastries and
Other Raised Baked Goods

These all contain high amounts of sugar. Sugar increases weight, energy dips, and hunger, and decreases your immune response to infections, cancer, and injuries. A high sugar diet will also contribute to blood-sugar imbalances and an increased risk of diabetes.

Processed and Smoked Meats

Deli meats, sausages, and smoked meats contain high amounts of salt, as well as preservatives, colorings, and nitrates. These chemicals promote heart disease and cancer and need to be avoided.

Fruit Juices and Soda

These all contain high amounts of sugar. Canned, bottled, and frozen juices, as well as all sodas, need to be avoided. Freshly squeezed fruit juice is fine.

What Now?

In summary, your meals should consist of vegetables, fruit, healthy fats and oils, and lean protein. Ideally half of your plate should be vegetables and the other half should be a combination of lean protein, healthy fats and oils, cooked legumes, and/or gluten-free whole grains.

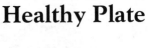

Healthy Plate

- Fresh Vegetables

- Healthy Fats and Oils, Lean Protein and Whole Grains/Legumes

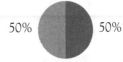

50%   50%

Include Foundation Supplements

I believe that everyone can benefit from three foundational supplements: a high-quality multivitamin, omega-3 fatty acids, and vitamin D. They all play such important roles and we really cannot afford to have deficient levels in any of them.

High-Quality Multivitamin

A high-quality multivitamin is important to supply your body with the nutrients that you may not be getting in your diet. I believe that, no matter how healthy we eat, we are still at risk of having some deficiencies because of overused and nutrient-depleted soil, and the abundant use of pesticides and herbicides.

Pesticides and herbicides protect fruits and vegetables from disease, but by doing this, the fruits and vegetables do not have to produce as much of their own protectants and phytonutrients. But it is these phytonutrients that supply us with powerful antioxidants, such as carotenoids, flavonoids, and ellagic acid, and function to fight particular cancers, decrease inflammation, and prevent allergies. It is important to have enough of these phytonutrients in our diet to prevent chronic disease and illness.

Soil conditions are the other big influence on the amount of phytonutrients a plant contains. Modern farming practices now allow for soil and fields to be used multiple times in a row for crop production. However, the overuse of these fields results in the soil being constantly stripped of its nutrients (phosphorus, zinc, magnesium, zinc, selenium, etc.) and not having the time to replenish. So the crops grown in these stripped fields are not able to uptake as many of the nutrients as they would have in the past, simply because those nutrients are not present in the soil.

Omega-3 Fatty Acids

Omega-3 fatty acids are very important to have in our diet because our bodies are unable to produce them on their own. They are crucial for optimal health and illness prevention. Omega-3s are essential for optimal brain function, nerve cell transmission, and cell membrane structure and function. They decrease inflammation and blood clotting and promote hormone synthesis. Omega-3s are found in high concentrations in fatty fish, flaxseed, and chia seeds, as well as kelp and walnuts. It is best to aim for at least two grams of omega-3 fatty acids per day.

Vitamin D3

Vitamin D is a powerful antioxidant, anti-cancer, and bone promoter. It helps regulate our immune system, promotes hormone synthesis, and increases mood. I test all of my clients for vitamin D3, and only about 10 percent of them have optimal levels. This decreased level of vitamin D increases the risk of immune disorders, poor mood, particular cancers, and osteoporosis.

The primary source of vitamin D is from sunlight; however, cod liver oil, halibut liver oil, and fatty fish also contain vitamin D. In order to get enough vitamin D from sunlight, you should be in the sun for at least 25 to 30 minutes every day with face, chest, and arms exposed.

Avoid Food Sensitivities

I also recommend being tested for food sensitivities. If you have unknown food sensitivities that you are eating on a daily basis, you will have increased inflammation in your body, possibly resulting in gas and abdominal bloating, acne, eczema, weight gain, migraine headaches, and/or fatigue. If you experience any of these symptoms, I highly suggest food-sensitivity testing.

Food-sensitivity testing is different from food-allergy testing in that food-allergy testing most often involves an allergist's skin-prick test. The allergist is testing if you have an allergic reaction instead of a sensitivity. Allergic reactions can present themselves as hives, eczema, breathing difficulties, and anaphylaxis, and generally involve the IgE antibody and histamine release. People with food allergies typically present with symptoms within a few minutes to a few hours after eating the allergic food.

Food sensitivities, on the other hand, involve the IgG antibody and often do not show symptoms for at least 2 to 48 hours later. The symptoms are more generalized and often hard to trace back to a particular food. This is why it is important to actually get a food-sensitivity test.

Helpful Tips

In order to make this diet transition easier for you, try making extras at dinner and save the leftovers for lunch the next day. See the "Recipe Collection" section for more ideas and recipes. If the diet described here is a dramatic change for you, your body may require a couple of weeks to adapt. Because this program is in part a detoxification program, you may feel tired for the first week or so, but keep with it. It will pay off in the end!

After about three weeks, you will begin to feel much better than you did before. And you will start to see your body, energy, weight, and mood change for good!

CHAPTER 7

Natural Solutions for Estrogen Excess: PMS, Irritability, and Weight Gain

E STROGEN IMBALANCES can arise from various factors. Nutritional deficiencies, environmental toxicity, slow liver detoxification, progesterone deficiency, aging, and stress can all contribute to estrogen imbalances. But with the proper support, your estrogen levels can be restored and maintained at optimal levels.

As I mentioned in the previous chapters, estrogen excess is a condition that I am seeing more and more often. Our environment is filled with xenoestrogens, chemicals that mimic estrogen in our body. These xenoestrogens are readily found in different plastics, cleaning supplies, cosmetics, water, and meat and dairy products. They build up in our bodies, causing abnormally high levels of estrogen and symptoms associated with estrogen excess. Estrogen excess often results in a relative progesterone deficiency, so both estrogen excess and progesterone deficiency have a similar symptom picture. The most common symptoms associated with estrogen excess are the typical PMS symptoms of breast tenderness, irritability, and heavy menstrual bleeding. Women with higher estrogen levels are also at higher risk of developing fibrocystic breasts, uterine fibroids, and ovarian cysts.

With estrogen excess, the goal is to improve your body's detoxification, avoid any further sources of xenoestrogens, and counterbalance with progesterone.

The diagram on the following page shows our liver detoxification pathways. This liver detox system is responsible for detoxifying our bodies from any harmful substances, as well as excess hormones such as estrogen. In the diagram you can see that many different vitamins are needed for this to happen, so it is important to ensure optimal levels of these nutrients.

Liver Detoxification

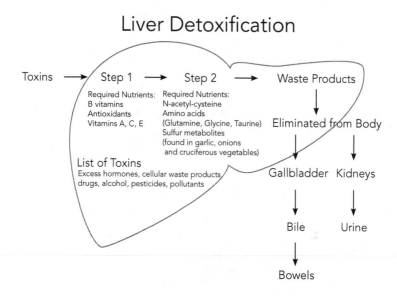

Step 1: Diet Support

In addition to the dietary guidelines outlined in the chapter "Nutrition for Happy Hormones," women with estrogen excess may benefit from extra fiber and lower amounts of sugar, caffeine, and alcohol.

Increase Fiber

Fiber binds up excess estrogen in the gastrointestinal (GI) tract and excretes it out of the body. It has been shown that women with a diet higher in fiber have less estrogen excess-related symptoms, such as irritability, breast tenderness, and bloating.

Decrease Alcohol and Caffeine

Alcohol, caffeine, and estrogen are all metabolized in the liver. If our liver is busy detoxing the caffeine and alcohol, it doesn't leave as much time or energy for estrogen detoxification. So, if you have estrogen excess, it is important to avoid alcohol and caffeine as much as possible.

Decrease Sugar

Many studies have shown that women with diets high in sugar have more estrogen-excess symptoms than women with diets lower in sugar.

Step 2: Lifestyle Support

Healthy lifestyle choices are vital for optimal hormone balance. Adequate sleep, minimal stress, exercise, and avoidance of xenoestrogens are all important for balanced estrogen levels.

Avoidance of Xenoestrogens

The most important lifestyle change you can make is to avoid further exposure to xenoestrogens. Xenoestrogens are found in our food, water, personal hygiene products, and plastics.

Below is a table showing some of the common sources of xenoestrogens.

COMMON SOURCES OF XENOESTROGENS	
PCBs, BPA	Plastics
Cosmetics containing phthalates and parabens	Dairy products
Dry cleaning chemicals	Pesticides
Birth-control pills	Cleaning supplies

Organic Foods

Focus on organic foods as much as you can. Pesticides and herbicides are high in xenoestrogens and should be avoided as much as possible. If you are to purchase only a few organic items, I suggest focusing on organic, hormone-free animal meats and dairy products.

Filtered, Non-Bottled Water

It is recommended you drink filtered tap water instead of bottled water. Plastic water bottles contain many different chemicals, including xenoestrogens, which can seep into the bottled water. This leaching of chemicals is particularly bad when the bottle is heated or left for a long time before being drank.

Plastic Avoidance

Xenoestrogens are present not only in plastic water bottles, but also in food storage containers and plastic bags. It is best to store your food in stainless steel or glass containers whenever possible.

Cosmetics

Cosmetics are another huge source of xenoestrogens. Both estrogen and xenoestrogens are added into various cosmetics. It is best to use mineral-based cosmetics and/or ones with ingredients that you can pronounce and are familiar with.

Cleaning Supplies

Conventional cleaning supplies contain xenoestrogens. It is best to swap out these conventional products with a supply of green cleaners.

For more information on safer cosmetics and cleaning supplies, check out the Environmental Working Group (www.ewg.org).

Step 3: Nutritional Support

Nutritional support includes the vitamins essential for liver detoxification, as well as a couple of minerals known to decrease estrogen excess-related symptoms.

Calcium and Magnesium

Calcium and magnesium have been shown to be beneficial for women experiencing estrogen-excess symptoms of PMS. They decrease breast tenderness, water retention, migraines, and irritability.

Magnesium is found in high concentrations in Brazil nuts, almonds, pecans, cashews, Swiss chard, kidney beans, soybeans, brown rice, and rye.

Calcium is found in high concentrations in turnip greens, spinach, sardines, spinach, tofu, broccoli, collard greens, and dairy products.

Calcium	600 mg daily
Magnesium	300 mg daily

Indole-3-carbinol and Diindolylmethane

Indole-3-carbinol (I3C) is a compound found in high concentrations in cruciferous vegetables, including broccoli, cauliflower, Brussels sprouts, and cabbage. When ingested, I3C is converted to diindolylmethane (DIM), which is then absorbed in the intestines. DIM is the primary contributor to I3C's beneficial properties, selectively binding to estrogen receptors and acting as an estrogen antagonist.

I3C also promotes the metabolism of estrogen in the liver so it can be safely excreted out of the body.

Indole-3-carbinol/ Diindolylmethane	200 mg, 1–2 times daily

Vitamin B Complex

B vitamins, in particular B2, B3, B6, B9, and B12, are needed for liver detoxification. The liver is our primary detoxification organ and is the main way we metabolize excess hormones. B vitamins are found in high concentrations in fish, poultry, pork loin, beef, whole grains, and various nuts and seeds.

Vitamin B Complex	At least 30 mg of vitamin B1 and B2, 50 mg of B6, and at least 800 mcg of vitamin B9 and B12 daily

Vitamins A, C, and E

Vitamins A, C, and E are all strong antioxidants necessary for our liver detoxification. These vitamins also protect our cells from damage and can have a beneficial effect in nerve disorders, inflammatory diseases, and cancer. See the table below for the foods rich in these vitamins.

Vitamin	*Food Sources*
Vitamin A	Liver, collard greens, spirulina, spinach, carrots, sweet potato, papaya, apricots
Vitamin C	Acerola berries, bell peppers, guava, watermelon, broccoli, Brussels sprouts, kiwi
Vitamin E	Sunflower oil and seeds, almonds, pecans, sweet potato, tempeh, hazelnuts, flaxseed oil, wheat germ oil

Vitamin A	5000–10,000 IU daily*
Vitamin C	1,000 mg, 2–3 times daily
Vitamin E (Mixed Tocopherols)	400–800 IU daily

*Not to be taken when pregnant

Amino Acids

Amino acids are the building blocks of protein. They are necessary for our everyday metabolic processes, such as the production of hormones, neurotransmitters, and enzymes, as well as for detoxification and energy production. It is essential we have enough protein in our diets, whether we have hormonal imbalances or not.

The amino acids most important for helping our body rid itself of excess estrogen are glutamine, lysine, carnitine, taurine, and cysteine. These are found in high concentrations in animal products, such as poultry, fish, beef, and dairy.

Foundation Supplements

I believe that everyone can benefit from three foundational supplements: a high-quality multivitamin, omega-3 fatty acids, and vitamin D. A high-quality multivitamin should have the abovementioned vitamins and minerals in adequate amounts. I've thoroughly discussed the benefits of these supplements in the chapter "Nutrition for Happy Hormones," as I think they should be part of your daily diet.

Step 4: Herbal Support

Vitex agnus-castus
(Chaste-tree Berry)

Vitex is a commonly used herb for female hormonal imbalances. It is called a pituitary balancer as it directly affects the production and release of pituitary hormones. It is thought to increase the production of luteinizing hormone, while inhibiting the release of follicle-stimulating hormone. This action favors progesterone production relative to estrogen. Vitex has been used effectively to decrease PMS symptoms, decrease the risk of miscarriage, promote regular menstrual cycles, and decrease the growth of breast and uterine fibroids.

Chaste-tree Berry (**Standardized Extract**)	200 mg, 1–2 times daily

Evening Primrose Oil

Evening primrose oil is great for estrogen-excess symptoms if there is a corresponding progesterone deficiency. Women supplemented with evening primrose oil during the second half of their menstrual cycle show marked improvements in the typical PMS symptoms of irritability, breast tenderness, and swelling, as well as decreased menstrual cramps.

Evening Primrose Oil	2–3 g daily

Silybum marianum
(Milk Thistle)

Milk thistle is mentioned here not because it directly influences hormones, but because of its action on the liver. Milk thistle helps stimulate the liver detoxification pathways and can actually protect the liver from some of the harmful toxins it comes in contact with. By promoting liver detoxification, milk thistle helps your body metabolize excess estrogens.

Milk Thistle (Silymarin Standardized Extract)	160 mg, 1–2 times daily

Taraxacum officinalis
(Dandelion Root)

Dandelion root, like milk thistle, works to promote liver detoxification and aids in the metabolism of excess estrogens. If we have slow liver detoxification, our estrogen levels can build up and cause estrogen excess-related symptoms.

Dandelion (Dried Root)	2 g daily

Step 5: Homeopathic Remedies

There are a variety of homeopathic remedies that people with an estrogen excess could benefit from. Please see my recommended homeopathic remedies in the Appendix.

Step 6: Hormone Replacement Support

In some cases, bioidentical progesterone support may be indicated. As mentioned before, estrogen excess is often associated with a relative progesterone deficiency. So, by supporting progesterone levels, we can counterbalance the excess estrogen. There are two types of progesterone hormone replacement: bioidentical and nonbioidentical (synthetic). As you will read in "Hormone Replacement Therapy" in the Appendix, bioidentical progesterone is better, safer, and, in my opinion, the only choice. If you are still menstruating, it is best to supplement with bioidentical progesterone only during the second phase of your menstrual cycle, as that is the time your progesterone levels are naturally increasing.

Prescription

Bioidentical progesterone is available in a few different forms: transdermal, oral, and sublingual (under the tongue).

20 to 30 mg of bioidentical progesterone in a transdermal cream or 100 to 200 mg in an oral pill form has been shown to significantly improve estrogen excess and progesterone deficiency symptoms.

BIOIDENTICAL PROGESTERONE REPLACEMENT	
Progesterone	Compounded bioidentical progesterone available in individualized doses as transdermal creams, oral formulations, or sublingual lozenges
Prometrium®	Brand name for bioidentical progesterone; oral formulation available in predetermined dosages only

Case Example: Paula, Age 33

Symptoms:
Paula came to my office with complaints of severe PMS. She said that, during the 10 days prior to her menstrual period, her breasts would swell and become tender, and she would get extremely depressed and irritable to the point of wanting to divorce her husband. Her husband actually kept track of her menstrual period so he would know when he needed to tread lightly. She had an extremely stressful childhood, and now worked in a high-stress job that left her exhausted every day. In addition to the PMS symptoms, Paula was also having a lot of digestive problems with gas, bloating, and constipation.

Diagnosis:
Based on Paula's symptoms picture and lab results, she was experiencing estrogen excess with a relative progesterone deficiency, accompanied by low vitamin D and cortisol. I also ran a food-sensitivity test, which showed sensitivities to gluten, wheat, eggs, and yeast.

Treatment:
I started Paula on bioidentical cortisol and progesterone, along with omega-3s, a high-quality multivitamin, vitamin D, indole-3-carbinol, and a supplement to stop the over-growth of intestinal yeast (candida). I also recommended she fully avoid her food sensitivities.

Results:

After six weeks, Paula's gastrointestinal symptoms were completely resolved, except when she would eat one of her food sensitivities. Her mood and energy were improved, along with a lessening of her PMS symptoms.

I checked in with her another eight weeks later and she was still doing well. After three months of treatment, her PMS was significantly improved, with no breast swelling or tenderness and a marked improvement in mood. Her husband was also happy with the progress. Since Paula was doing so much better, we discontinued the bioidentical cortisol and progesterone after three months to see if her hormonal system was rested enough to pick up the slack and keep her at optimal levels. Six weeks after stopping the bioidentical hormones, she was still doing great.

CHAPTER 8

Natural Solutions for Estrogen Deficiency: Hot Flashes, Insomnia, and Dryness

E STROGEN DEFICIENCY is most often seen in post-menopausal women. Throughout menopause the ovaries slowly decrease their estrogen production, and it is up to our adrenal glands to take over. However, usually by this point in our lives, our adrenal glands are tired and having a hard enough time just producing enough cortisol. As a result, our estrogen levels that are naturally already declining can decline even quicker, leading to the typical menopause symptoms. With estrogen deficiency, the goal is to support natural estrogen production, while decreasing the side effects of low estrogen.

Step 1: Diet Support

In addition to the dietary guidelines outlined in the chapter "Nutrition for Happy Hormones," women with estrogen deficiency may benefit from lower amounts of sugar, caffeine, spicy foods, and alcohol.

Avoid Spicy Foods

Spicy foods have been shown to trigger hot flashes. Just by removing spicy foods from your diet, you will notice a decrease in the frequency of hot flashes.

Decrease Alcohol and Caffeine

Alcohol and caffeine, like spicy foods, also trigger hot flashes and night sweats. But, in addition to this, increased consumption of caffeine is correlated with lower estrogen levels in premenopausal women.

Include Whole Soy in Moderation

Soy is very controversial. My clients often ask my opinion on soy: should they eat it or should they avoid it? My recommendation is to include whole soy (organic tofu, soybeans, and/or tempeh) in your diet, but in moderation: no more than two times per week. Soy contains estrogen-modulating compounds, which help promote your body's estrogen production and/or estrogen effects. The studies surrounding the effect of soy on estrogen levels show conflicting results, but what we do know is that Asian women who consume whole and fermented soy have reduced menopausal symptoms of hot flashes, night sweats, and osteoporosis. Processed soy products (such as soy yogurt, milk, and cheese) often contain additives and preservatives and are not recommended. In addition, I am seeing more and more patients with sensitivities to soy, so before increasing soy in your diet, I recommend you get tested for food sensitivities.

Step 2: Lifestyle Support

Healthy lifestyle choices are vital for optimal hormone balance. Adequate sleep, minimal stress, routine, healthy eating, and exercise are all important for optimal estrogen levels.

Decrease Stress

Stress can actually lead to decreased estrogen levels. When we experience stress, our body can shunt the hormone pathways toward cortisol production and away from progesterone and estrogen production. Because of this, it is important to find ways in which you can decrease your stress. Think of the areas in your life that cause you the most stress and brainstorm about what you can do to decrease this. It may be looking for a new job, slowing down on nonpersonal and work commitments, or spending more time doing things you enjoy.

Weight-Bearing Exercise

Exercise is another important aspect to consider. Women with low estrogen levels have an increased risk of osteoporosis. Estrogen is needed to block the breakdown of bone, so if our estrogen levels decrease, so does our ability to maintain our bone mass. Weight-bearing exercise, such as walking and lifting weights, helps maintain and even restore bone mass.

Routine

Establishing a routine is important for overall hormonal balance. Each day of the week, try to wake up and go to bed at the same time, and eat your meals at the same times. By establishing a regular routine, your stress response will decrease, your metabolism will balance out, and you will feel an increase in energy and mood.

Step 3: Nutritional Support

The supplements used in estrogen deficiency focus on adrenal function and bone health. As our estrogen levels decrease, we begin to lose calcium from our bones, so we need to ensure we are getting enough calcium and vitamins D and K to promote and maintain bone health.

Vitamins C and E

Vitamins C and E are useful during menopause because they benefit the adrenal glands. As we know, the adrenal glands are responsible for producing the majority of sex hormones, including estrogen, after menopause. We need to nourish the adrenal glands so they can effectively cope with this increased demand. See the table below for foods high in vitamins C and E.

Vitamin	Food Sources
Vitamin C	Acerola berries, bell peppers, guava, watermelon, broccoli, Brussels sprouts, kiwi
Vitamin E	Sunflower oil and seeds, almonds, pecans, sweet potato, tempeh, hazelnuts, flaxseed oil, wheat-germ oil

Vitamin C	1,000 mg, 2–3 times daily
Vitamin E	400–800 IU daily

Calcium

Calcium plays an important role in maintaining bone mass in postmenopausal women. As our estrogen levels decline, our bones begin to lose calcium at a faster rate. This calcium loss is what can eventually lead to osteopenia and osteoporosis in postmenopausal women. Therefore, it is important to ensure you are getting enough calcium. Great sources of calcium include turnip greens, spinach, sardines, spinach, tofu, broccoli, collard greens, and dairy products.

Calcium Citrate	400 mg, twice daily

Vitamin D

Vitamin D is needed to maintain serum calcium concentrations. It increases calcium levels by promoting its absorption in the intestines. If serum calcium levels drop, your body will start drawing it out of your bone tissue to compensate. Over time this can lead to osteoporosis. Without sufficient vitamin D, as little as 10 to 15 percent of dietary calcium is absorbed.

Vitamin D is not only important for bone health. It has been shown to protect against breast and colon cancer, elevate mood, and balance our immune system.

Our primary source of vitamin D is through sun exposure. It is estimated that 20 minutes of sun exposure, with face and arms exposed, will produce about 200 IU of vitamin D. There are not many nonfortified food sources of vitamin D other than oily fish, such as sardines, herring, mackerel, halibut, and cod liver oil.

Vitamin D3	2,000 IU daily*

Dose may vary, depending on blood serum levels

Vitamin K2

Vitamin K2, like calcium and vitamin D, is important for maintaining bone mass. It allows calcium ions to bind to bone so bone calcification can occur. Sources of vitamin K include turnip greens, broccoli, cabbage, beef liver, and green tea.

Vitamin K2	5–10 mg daily*

*Can interfere with the anticlotting effects of blood thinners, warfarin, and Coumadin®

Foundation Supplements

I believe that everyone can benefit from three foundational supplements: a high-quality multivitamin, omega-3 fatty acids, and vitamin D. A high-quality multivitamin should have the abovementioned vitamins and minerals in adequate amounts. I've thoroughly discussed the benefits of these supplements in the chapter "Nutrition for Happy Hormones," as I think they should be part of your daily diet.

Step 4: Herbal Support

Cimicifuga racemosa
(Black Cohosh)

Black cohosh is a well-known herb in the treatment of meno-pausal symptoms. Many women report decreased severity and frequency of hot flashes, night sweats, and irritability when taking black cohosh. How black cohosh accomplishes this is still a bit of a mystery. Early research showed it was a phytoestrogen capable of supporting our body's production of estrogen and suppressing the surge of luteinizing hormone. However, new research is showing otherwise. Despite this lack of understanding, we do know that it makes a significant difference in menopausal symptoms.

Black Cohosh	200–400 mg daily

Medicago sativa
(Alfalfa)

Alfalfa is considered to be a phytoestrogen, an herb capable of promoting estrogen production and/or estrogenic effects in the body. It has been shown to improve the symptoms associated with estrogen deficiency and menopause.

Alfalfa (Dried)	3–6 g daily

Tribulus terrestris
(Tribulus)

Tribulus is a not a well-known herb, but it is quite effective at modulating estrogen levels and improving many symptoms associated with estrogen deficiency and menopause. It is gaining popularity as a fertility herb, as it has been shown to act as an ovarian stimulant and normalize ovulation.

Tribulus (**Standardized Extract**)	200–400 mg daily

Step 5: Homeopathic Remedies

There are a variety of homeopathic remedies that people with an estrogen deficiency could benefit from. Please see my recommended homeopathic remedies in the Appendix.

Step 6: Hormone Replacement Support

Sometimes bioidentical hormone replacement may be necessary to restore optimal estrogen levels. By replacing estrogen, menopausal symptoms, such as hot flashes, vaginal dryness, night sweats, irritability, and dry skin and eyes, will significantly improve. Besides improving the symptoms associated with menopause, estrogen replacement can also decrease your risk of future cardiovascular disease and help maintain your memory and bone and muscle mass.

Estrogen replacement is covered in more detail in "Hormone Replacement Therapy" in the Appendix.

Bioidentical estrogen is available in a few different formulas and application methods.

BIOIDENTICAL ESTROGEN FORMULATIONS	
Estradiol	Tri-estrogen
Estriol	Estrace®
Bi-estrogen	Gynodiol®

Case Example: Nina, Age 59

Symptoms:

Nina came to my practice one year after her menopausal symptoms had started. She was hoping they would eventually go away, but was getting exhausted waiting for that to happen. She complained of poor sleep, hot flashes, irritability, and difficulty remembering some very basic things.

Diagnosis:

Based on Nina's symptom picture and lab results, I determined she was suffering from low estrogen and progesterone levels, as well as suboptimal thyroid function.

Treatment:

I prescribed Nina bioidentical bi-estrogen, oral progesterone (to help with sleep), and a multivitamin designed for menopausal women to ensure optimal vitamin D, K2, calcium, and some other trace minerals important for bone health. I also suggested she take omega-3s to help with her cognitive function and dry skin. In terms of dietary recommendations, I asked her to avoid caffeine and spicy foods.

Results:

After six weeks, Nina's hot flashes were completely resolved. Her energy and sleep were both greatly improved. At this point, she didn't notice much improvement with her memory, so we decided to check in again in another six weeks.

At that next appointment, Nina was still sleeping well, with no recurrence of hot flashes. She was feeling great. She thought her memory was improving little by little, so we continued with the same treatment program, expecting to see gradual improvement in her memory. We continued to monitor her energy and thyroid values to see if they would improve with the treatment program, and sure enough, they came into optimal range.

CHAPTER 9

Natural Solutions for Progesterone Deficiency: Infertility, Irritability, PMS, and Insomnia

PROGESTERONE IMBALANCES can arise from various factors. Nutritional deficiencies, estrogen excess, slow liver detoxification, and stress can all contribute to progesterone deficiency. But with proper support, your progesterone levels can be restored and maintained at optimal levels.

When supporting progesterone, it is important to mimic our body's natural production and release. You can see in the figure on the following page how progesterone levels change throughout the menstrual cycle. In premenopausal women, it's best to support progesterone only during the second phase of the menstrual cycle (from day 14 to day 28) because this is when your progesterone levels are normally increasing. However, since postmenopausal women no longer have a regular menstrual cycle, progesterone support can be given throughout the entire menstrual cycle. If progesterone is cycled in postmenopausal women, menstrual bleeding can occur within a couple of days of stopping the progesterone.

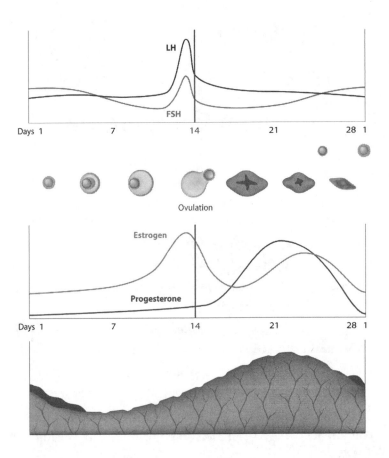

Step 1: Diet Support

In addition to the dietary guidelines outlined in the chapter "Nutrition for Happy Hormones," women with progesterone deficiency may benefit from extra fiber and lower amounts of sugar, caffeine, and alcohol.

Increase Fiber

Fiber binds up excess estrogen in the GI tract and excretes it out of the body. And as you read earlier, excess estrogen contributes to a relative progesterone deficiency. It has been shown that women with a diet higher in fiber have less progesterone deficiency-related symptoms, such as irritability, breast tenderness, and bloating.

Decrease Alcohol and Caffeine

Alcohol, caffeine, and estrogen are all metabolized in the liver. If our liver is busy detoxing the caffeine and alcohol, it doesn't leave as much time or energy for estrogen detoxification. In this way, moderate consumption of alcohol and caffeine can lead to an overall estrogen excess and progesterone deficiency.

Decrease Sugar

Many studies have shown that women with diets high in sugar and foods containing sugar have more progesterone deficiency symptoms than women with diets lower in sugar.

Step 2: Lifestyle Support

Healthy lifestyle choices are vital for optimal hormone balance. Adequate sleep, minimal stress, routine, healthy eating, and exercise are all important for optimal progesterone levels.

Decrease Stress

Stress can actually decrease progesterone levels. When there is excess stress, there is an increased need for cortisol. In order to get this extra cortisol, our body shunts the hormone pathways away from progesterone and estrogen production in favor of cortisol production. This results in lower progesterone levels. So, it is important to find ways in which you can decrease your stress. Think of the areas in your life that cause you the most stress and brainstorm what you can do to decrease this. It may be looking for a new job, slowing down on nonpersonal and work commitments, or spending more time doing things you enjoy.

Exercise

Exercise is another important aspect to consider. Women with low progesterone levels often feel depressed and fatigued. Moderate exercise increases our metabolism and the release of natural endorphins, leading to increased energy and happier thoughts and feelings.

Routine

Establishing a routine is important for overall hormonal balance. Each day of the week, try to wake up and go to bed at the same time, and eat your meals at the same times. By establishing a regular routine, your stress response will decrease, your metabolism will balance out, and you will feel an increase in energy and mood.

Step 3: Nutritional Support

Many women notice an improvement in their progesterone deficiency symptoms just by increasing specific vitamins and minerals. These nutrients include magnesium, calcium, vitamin B6, and essential fatty acids.

Magnesium

Magnesium has been shown to be beneficial for progesterone-deficient women. It decreases the symptoms of breast tenderness, water retention, migraines, and irritability. Women with progesterone-deficiency symptoms have been shown to have lower levels of magnesium in their red blood cells compared to women with optimal progesterone levels. Magnesium can be found in high concentrations in Brazil nuts, almonds, pecans, cashews, Swiss chard, kidney beans, soybeans, brown rice, and rye.

Magnesium (**Elemental or Citrate**)	400 mg, twice daily

Calcium

Calcium, like magnesium, has been shown to decrease the symptoms associated with progesterone deficiency. In a few different studies, women supplemented with calcium showed a marked improvement in mood, breast swelling and tenderness, and overall water retention. Calcium is found in high concentrations in turnip greens, spinach, sardines, spinach, tofu, broccoli, collard greens, and dairy products.

Calcium Citrate	600 mg daily

Vitamin B6

Vitamin B6 has been associated with improving progesterone deficiency-related symptoms, such as irritability, low mood, fatigue, and anxiety. It also contributes to increased levels of our happy neurotransmitters, dopamine and serotonin. Vitamin B6 can be found in many different species of fish, poultry, pork loin, bran cereal, bananas, watermelon, avocado, and sunflower seeds.

Vitamin B6	50 mg, twice daily

Evening Primrose Oil

Evening primrose oil has been associated with a decrease in progesterone deficiency-related symptoms. It contains an essential fatty acid called gamma linolenic acid, known to

balance hormones and decrease inflammation. Women supplemented with evening primrose oil during the second half
of their menstrual cycle show marked improvements in the
typical PMS symptoms of irritability and breast tenderness
and swelling, as well as decreased menstrual cramps.

Evening Primrose Oil	2–3 g daily

Foundation Supplements

I believe that everyone can benefit from three foundational supplements: a high-quality multivitamin, omega-3
fatty acids, and vitamin D. A high-quality multivitamin
should have the abovementioned vitamins and minerals
in adequate amounts. I've thoroughly discussed the benefits of these supplements in the chapter "Nutrition for
Happy Hormones," as I think they should be part of your
daily diet.

Step 4: Herbal Support

Vitex agnus-castus
(Chaste-tree Berry)

Vitex is a commonly used herb for female hormonal imbalances. It is called a pituitary balancer, as it affects the production and release of various pituitary hormones. It is thought
to increase the production of luteinizing hormone, while
inhibiting the release of follicle-stimulating hormone. This

action promotes the production of progesterone. Vitex has been used effectively to decrease PMS symptoms, decrease the risk of miscarriage, promote regular menstrual cycles, and decrease the growth of breast and uterine fibroids.

Chaste-tree Berry (Standardized Extract)	200 mg, twice daily

Smilax ornata *(Sarsaparilla)*

Smilax is used for a variety of hormonal imbalances. It is thought to have progesteronic actions and is best used to support the luteal phase of the menstrual cycle.

Sarsaparilla	1–2 g daily

Taraxacum officinalis *(Dandelion Root)*

Taraxacum does not directly influence hormone levels, but instead works to promote liver detoxification. If we have slow liver detoxification, our estrogen levels can build up, resulting in a relative estrogen excess and progesterone deficiency.

Dandelion (Dried Root)	2 g daily

A note about wild yam (*Dioscorea villosa*): it is a common belief that wild yam increases progesterone levels. However, this is not the case. Natural bioidentical progesterone is synthesized from wild yam, but only after it has been manipulated in a laboratory. Wild yam does contain progesterone precursors; however, we are unable to convert those precursors into actual progesterone. So, if you are taking wild yam in hopes of increasing your progesterone levels, it won't do you much good.

Step 5: Homeopathic Remedies

There are a variety of homeopathic remedies that people with a progesterone deficiency could benefit from. Please see my recommended homeopathic remedies in the Appendix.

Step 6: Hormone Replacement Support

In some cases, hormone replacement may be necessary to restore optimal progesterone levels. By replacing progesterone, symptoms of insomnia, PMS, depression, and breast tenderness and swelling will significantly improve. There are two types of progesterone hormone replacement: bioidentical and nonbioidentical (synthetic). Bioidentical progesterone is the better, safer choice (and, in my opinion, the only choice). If you are menstruating, it is best to supplement with bioidentical progesterone only during the second phase of your menstrual cycle, as that is the time when your progesterone levels are naturally increasing. If you no longer menstruate, you can supplement with bioidentical progesterone throughout the entire month.

Bioidentical progesterone is available in a few different forms: transdermal, oral, and sublingual (under the tongue). Twenty to 30 mg of bioidentical progesterone in a transdermal cream or 100 to 200 mg in an oral pill form have been shown to significantly improve progesterone-deficiency symptoms. Progesterone replacement is covered in more detail in the "Hormone Replacement Therapy" section in the Appendix.

BIOIDENTICAL PROGESTERONE REPLACEMENT	
Progesterone	Compounded bioidentical progesterone available in individualized doses as transdermal creams, oral formulation, or sublingual lozenges
Prometrium®	Brand name for bioidentical progesterone; oral formulation available only in predetermined dosages

Case Example: Mary, Age 42

Symptoms:
When I first met Mary, she was experiencing chronic tiredness. She had just taken a year off work to see if that would help, but according to her, it didn't make a difference. She explained that her and her husband had been trying to conceive for the past eight months with little success. During those eight months, she conceived once, but had a miscarriage eight weeks later.

Diagnosis:
After running a few lab tests, I confirmed that Mary had both cortisol and progesterone deficiency. There was also an underlying iron, vitamin B12, and vitamin D deficiency.

Treatment:
I started Mary on adrenal extracts, ashwagandha, omega-3s, iron, and a high-quality vitamin containing vitamins C and E. I also prescribed her a bioidentical progesterone cream to take from days 14 to 28 of her menstrual cycle. I talked with her about the importance of eating a diet rich in vegetables, healthy oils, and lean protein.

Results:
After six weeks, Mary noticed significant improvements in her energy levels. She went from a 5 of 10 to an 8 of 10. She

also said she noticed an improvement in her concentration and mood. I advised her to keep on the treatment program for another three months before discontinuing the progesterone cream. Four months down the road, Mary conceived and gave birth to a healthy boy nine months later.

CHAPTER 10

Natural Solutions for Cortisol Excess: Stress, Anxiety, and Irritability

CORTISOL IMBALANCE usually starts off as an excess, and then can either quickly or slowly progress into adrenal fatigue and cortisol deficiency. Some people can function with high cortisol levels for their entire life without progressing into adrenal fatigue, whereas others can rapidly progress into adrenal fatigue after an illness or a difficult life change.

With the proper support, your adrenal function can be restored and your cortisol levels maintained at optimal levels. This support most often includes nutritional support, lifestyle modifications, and a variety of herbs or supplements.

Cortisol excess is most often associated with the stress response. However, sometimes cortisol excess can be caused by a disorder called Cushing's syndrome or Cushing's disease. If your cortisol levels are extremely high, it is recommended you speak with your physician to rule out Cushing's. Symptoms of cortisol excess include anxiety, irritability, nervousness, difficulty sleeping, high blood pressure, and even weight gain.

Step 1: Diet Support

In addition to the dietary guidelines outlined in the chapter "Nutrition for Happy Hormones," people with excess cortisol benefit from a diet high in protein and low in starch and sugar. Caffeine and other stimulants should also be avoided.

Increase Protein

Excess cortisol can actually cause higher blood-sugar levels, predisposing you to an increased risk of insulin resistance and diabetes. A diet low in protein and high in starchy carbohydrates will amplify this imbalance because starchy carbohydrates are rapidly broken down into sugar in our bodies. So incorporate protein with every meal to help stabilize your blood sugar and decrease your risk of insulin resistance and diabetes. Some examples of foods high in protein include nuts and seeds, poultry, beef, fish, and nut butters.

Decrease Caffeine and Other Stimulants

Caffeine and other stimulants trigger the stress response in our bodies, and if you already have excess cortisol levels, these will only leave you feeling more stressed and anxious. In addition, your adrenal glands will have to produce even more cortisol, which may eventually leave them tired and unable to respond to stress adequately in the future.

Decrease Sugar

Excess cortisol leads to increased blood-sugar levels and an increased risk for insulin resistance and diabetes. To keep your blood sugar at an optimal level, it is best to avoid sugar in your diet. Even if you don't have excess cortisol levels, it is still recommended to avoid sugar, as it decreases our immune function and contributes to obesity and heart disease.

Step 2: Lifestyle Support

Healthy lifestyle choices are vital for optimal hormone balance. Adequate sleep, minimal stress, routine, healthy eating, and exercise are all important for balancing cortisol.

Decrease Stress

It is important to find ways in which you can decrease your stress. When you are stressed, your body goes into fight-or-flight mode, shutting down the digestive and immune systems, while increasing blood-sugar levels. Eventually this can lead to health problems, such as high blood pressure, obesity, digestive complaints, and adrenal fatigue. Think of the areas in your life that cause you the most stress and brainstorm what you can do to decrease this. It may be looking for a new job, slowing down on nonpersonal and work commitments, and/or spending more time doing things you enjoy.

Moderate Exercise

Exercise is another important aspect to consider. Exercise not only relieves stress, but also increases our metabolism and the release of natural endorphins, leading to increased energy and happier thoughts and feelings. However, intense exercise actually triggers the stress response, so if you already have excess cortisol levels, it is important to focus on light to moderate exercise. People with excess cortisol respond very well to yoga and meditation, as both of these significantly decrease stress.

Sufficient Sleep

Sufficient sleep is very important. You need a good night's rest to function at an optimal level the next day and adequately respond to stress. Many people with high cortisol have a hard time falling asleep at night because they are a bit anxious. If this is the case with you, think about skullcap, passionflower, and a meditation session before bed.

Routine

Establishing a routine is important for overall hormonal balance. Each day of the week, try to wake up and go to bed at the same time, and eat your meals at the same times. By establishing a regular routine, your stress response will decrease, your metabolism will balance out, and you will feel an increase in energy and mood.

Step 3: Nutritional Support

There are a few different vitamins necessary for your adrenal glands' production of cortisol, norepinephrine, and epinephrine in response to stress. These include vitamin C, vitamin E, vitamin B5, and vitamin B6.

Vitamin C

Vitamin C must be present in optimal levels in order for your adrenal glands to efficiently cope with stress. It is a necessary cofactor for the actual production of cortisol, norepinephrine, and epinephrine. Vitamin C is also a strong antioxidant, cancer preventative, and collagen generator. It can be found in high concentrations in acerola berries, guava, red chili peppers, green and sweet bell peppers, grapefruit, watermelon, kiwi, Brussels sprouts, cauliflower, and broccoli.

Vitamin C	1,000 mg, 2–3 times daily

Vitamin E

Vitamin E, like vitamin C, plays an important role in the production of cortisol. The highest concentrations of vitamin E are found in the adrenal glands and pituitary gland. Besides its role in the production of cortisol, vitamin E is also a strong antioxidant and nerve and muscle protectant.

Vitamin E is found in high concentrations in almonds, hazelnuts, sunflower seeds, pecans, flaxseed oil, sunflower and safflower oil, sweet potatoes, and tempeh.

Vitamin E (Mixed Tocopherols)	800 IU daily

Vitamin B5

Vitamin B5 has been associated with optimal adrenal function during times of stress. It is needed for the synthesis of a few different steroid hormones, including cortisol. Research has shown that people with optimal levels of vitamin B5 have an increased ability to deal with stress. High concentrations of vitamin B5 can be found in chicken and beef liver, dark poultry meat, brewer's yeast, beef, eggs, and brown rice.

Vitamin B5	500 mg, twice daily

Foundation Supplements

I believe that everyone can benefit from three foundational supplements: a high-quality multivitamin, omega-3 fatty acids, and vitamin D. A high-quality multivitamin should have the abovementioned vitamins and minerals in adequate amounts. I've thoroughly discussed the benefits of these supplements in the chapter "Nutrition for Happy Hormones," as I think they should be part of your daily diet.

Step 4: Herbal Support

Withania somnifera
(Ashwagandha)

Ashwagandha is an extremely important herb for adrenal imbalances. It is considered an adrenal adaptogen, meaning it can bring adrenal function back into normal ranges. If cortisol levels are too high, ashwagandha will actually work to decrease cortisol production, thereby bringing cortisol levels back into normal range. Ashwagandha has been shown to increase energy, strength, and libido, as well as decrease inflammation.

Ashwagandha (Dried Root)	600 mg, twice daily

Eleutherococcus senticosus
(Siberian Ginseng)

Siberian ginseng, like ashwagandha, is an adrenal adaptogen. It is great in calming anxiety, increasing endurance and stamina, and improving mental fatigue. It is a great herb for both cortisol excess and deficiency.

Siberian Ginseng (Dried Root)	800 mg, twice daily

Passiflora incarnata
(Passionflower)

Passionflower is a strong anxiolytic that can reduce irritability, anxiety, and insomnia. It is an ideal herb for people with excess cortisol who experience sleep-onset and sleep-maintenance insomnia due to a stressed, busy mind.

Passionflower (Dried Aerial Parts)	500 mg, twice daily

Scutellaria lateriflora
(Skullcap)

Skullcap, like passionflower, is an anxiolytic herb. It decreases anxiety, emotional stress, and insomnia, making it an ideal herb for people experiencing stress and high cortisol levels. Skullcap is also great for tension headaches.

Skullcap (Dried Root)	600 mg, twice daily

Step 5: Homeopathic Remedies

There are a variety of homeopathic remedies that people with high cortisol could benefit from. Please see my recommended homeopathic remedies in the Appendix.

Step 6: Hormone Replacement Support

Hormone replacement therapy is not indicated for cortisol excess, unless there are accompanying hormonal deficiencies that need to be supported.

Case Example: Louise, Age 36

Symptoms:

As Louise walked into my office, I could already feel the stress emitting from her. She was coming to her appointment straight from work, where she was a paralegal with multiple deadlines and daily stress. She said that in the past year she was constantly sick with colds and flu, felt irritable, and had a hard time sleeping at night. She said that, since she was so busy with work, she didn't have time to cook, exercise, or do anything for herself.

Diagnosis:

After speaking with her and ordering some lab tests, it turned out she was in a cortisol-excess state with an underlying iron and vitamin D deficiency.

Treatment:

I first spoke with Louise about decreasing her stress. I asked her to think of everything in her life that caused her stress and brainstorm how she could decrease this. In addition, I asked her to go for a 20-minute walk every day in the park next to her house and recommended that she designate two hours every Sunday to prepare meals for the next week. I mentioned the importance of decreasing stress, establishing a routine, and avoiding any stimulants, such as coffee and black tea. In terms of supplements, I prescribed her iron, vitamin D, omega-3, a good-quality multivitamin, and an ashwagandha and skullcap herbal formula to help modulate her adrenal stress response.

Results:

After three weeks, Louise said she was feeling much better. She had actually decided to leave her job and was currently looking for another job with a more positive environment. Her energy increased from 5 to 8 out of 10, and she was sleeping better. She said she could sleep at night now because she was no longer worrying about work. She had been walking every day in the park for the past two weeks and made some meals at home. She said she felt more calm and relaxed.

I checked in with her eight weeks later, and she was still doing well. She was keeping up with the walks, cooking on Sundays, and getting lots of sleep. Her energy was still up at an 8, and she hadn't been sick with a cold since our first appointment.

This case study really shows the affect of stress on our health and just how important it is to identify stressors and decrease them however you can.

CHAPTER 11

Natural Solutions for Cortisol Deficiency: Fatigue, Brain Fog, and Feeling Overwhelmed

C ORTISOL IMBALANCE usually starts off as an excess, and then can either slowly or quite quickly progress into adrenal fatigue and cortisol deficiency. Some people can function with high cortisol levels for their entire life without progressing into adrenal fatigue, whereas others can rapidly progress into adrenal fatigue after an illness or a difficult life change.

With the proper support, your adrenal function can be restored and your cortisol levels maintained at optimal levels. This support most often includes nutritional support, lifestyle modifications, and a variety of herbs or supplements.

Low cortisol and adrenal fatigue can be extremely debilitating for some people. The fatigue, feelings of being overwhelmed, low mood, and difficulty coping with stress can hinder daily performance, leading to difficulties at work and home. When looking at support for low cortisol levels, it is important to address your individual symptoms and lab results in order to choose an appropriate treatment program. The main goal of adrenal support is to decrease stress and nourish the adrenal glands so they can produce more cortisol themselves.

Step 1: Diet Support

In addition to the dietary guidelines outlined in the chapter "Nutrition for Happy Hormones," people with adrenal fatigue benefit from a diet high in protein and low in refined carbohydrates. Caffeine and other stimulants should also be avoided.

Increase Protein and Decrease Sugar

A higher protein diet will help stabilize your blood-sugar levels and increase energy. Try to incorporate protein with every meal. Some examples of foods high in protein include nuts and seeds, poultry, beef, fish, and nut butters.

Sugar tends to leave adrenally fatigued people feeling even more tired, so avoid sugar and foods containing sugar as much as possible.

Decrease Caffeine and Other Stimulants

Caffeine and other stimulants trigger the stress response in our bodies, so if you are already having a hard enough time dealing with your everyday stress, these will only add more fuel to the fire. You need to focus on decreasing stress from all sources: physical, mental/emotional, and dietary.

Step 2: Lifestyle Support

Healthy lifestyle choices are vital for optimal hormone balance. Adequate sleep, minimal stress, routine, healthy eating, and exercise are all important for balancing cortisol.

Decrease Stress

You are most likely suffering from adrenal fatigue and low cortisol levels because of high stress, so it is important to find ways in which you can decrease this. Your adrenal glands need to recover, and every little stress they have to deal with lengthens this recovery process. Think of the areas in your life that cause you the most stress and brainstorm what you can do to decrease this. It may be looking for a new job, slowing down on nonpersonal and work commitments, or spending more time doing things you enjoy and less time doing things you don't. Meditation is also a great way to decrease stress, and I recommend it for everyone with adrenal fatigue.

Exercise

Exercise is very healthy for us, but it is also a form of physical stress, and with adrenal fatigue, you are already having a hard enough time dealing with daily stressors. Because of this, I recommend exercising, but keeping it to the lighter exercises like yoga, pilates, walking, and light weight lifting. When you have adrenal fatigue, it is important to listen to your body and stop exercising when you feel tired. Also, if you feel exhausted after exercising either right after or the next day, this means you have done too much. Listen to your body and work yourself up slowly.

Routine

Establishing a routine is important for overall hormonal balance. Each day of the week, try to wake up and go to bed at the same time, and eat your meals at the same times. By establishing a regular routine, your stress response will decrease, your metabolism will balance out, and you will feel an increase in energy and mood.

Step 3: Nutritional Support

The same supplements useful for cortisol excess are also essential for adrenal fatigue and low cortisol levels. These vitamins focus on supporting and nourishing the adrenal glands, whether they are producing too much or too little cortisol. One important addition to the nutritional support for adrenal fatigue are adrenal glandulars.

Adrenal Glandulars and Extracts

Adrenal glandulars are adrenal supplements made up of actual adrenal gland tissue, usually from porcine or bovine (pig or cow) sources. They provide your adrenal glands with the raw materials they need during the recovery process. When adrenal glandulars are added to a treatment program, the adrenal fatigue improves at a quicker pace. But keep in mind that the recovery of the adrenal glands is not a fast process; it can take anywhere from six months to one year, but improvement is usually seen within the first few months.

Adrenal Cortex Extracts	250 mg, 2–3 times daily

Vitamin C

Vitamin C is critical for adrenal gland function and recovery. It is a necessary cofactor for the actual production of cortisol, norepinephrine, and epinephrine. Vitamin C is also a strong antioxidant, cancer preventative, and collagen generator. It can be found in high concentrations in acerola berries, guava, red chili peppers, green and sweet bell peppers, grapefruit, watermelon, kiwi, Brussels sprouts, cauliflower, and broccoli.

Vitamin C	1,000 mg, 2–3 times daily

Vitamin E

Vitamin E, like vitamin C, plays an important role in the production of cortisol. It must be at optimal levels in order for your adrenal glands to recover and restore their hormones. The highest concentrations of vitamin E are found in the adrenal glands and the pituitary gland. Besides its role in the production of cortisol, vitamin E is also a strong antioxidant and nerve and muscle protectant. Vitamin E is found in high concentrations in almonds, hazelnuts, sunflower seeds, pecans, flaxseed oil, sunflower and safflower oil, sweet potatoes, and tempeh.

Vitamin E (Mixed Tocopherols)	800 IU daily

Vitamin B5

Vitamin B5 is necessary for optimal adrenal function during times of stress. It is so essential for the synthesis of adrenal steroid hormones that, if there is a deficiency, your adrenal glands can actually shrink in size. High concentrations of vitamin B5 can be found in chicken and beef liver, dark poultry meat, brewer's yeast, beef, eggs, and brown rice.

Vitamin B5	500 mg, twice daily

Foundation Supplements

I believe that everyone can benefit from three foundational supplements: a high-quality multivitamin, omega-3 fatty acids, and vitamin D. A high-quality multivitamin should have the abovementioned vitamins and minerals in adequate amounts. I've thoroughly discussed the benefits of these supplements in the chapter "Nutrition for Happy Hormones," as I think they should be part of your daily diet.

Step 4: Herbal Support

Withania somnifera
(Ashwagandha)

Ashwagandha is an extremely important herb for adrenal imbalances. It is considered an adrenal adaptogen, meaning it can bring adrenal function back into normal ranges. If cortisol levels are too low, ashwagandha will actually work to increase cortisol production, thereby bringing cortisol levels back into normal range. Besides acting as an adrenal adaptogen, ashwagandha also increases energy, strength, endurance, and libido and decreases inflammation, making it particularly useful in inflammatory conditions, such as rheumatoid arthritis and osteoarthritis, both of which are commonly associated with adrenal fatigue.

Ashwagandha **(Dried Root)**	600 mg, twice daily

Eleutherococcus senticosus
(Siberian Ginseng)

Siberian ginseng, like ashwagandha, is an adrenal adaptogen. It improves mental concentration, sustains energy levels and endurance, and decreases irritability. It often has a very positive effect on mood. Siberian ginseng is also considered to be an immune-modulating herb, meaning it will strengthen the immune system so it is better able to fight off illness. People with adrenal fatigue often end up with cold after cold because of a weakened immune system, and Siberian ginseng is a great herb to finally put an end to that cold cycle.

Siberian Ginseng **(Dried Root)**	800 mg, twice daily

Glycyrrhiza glabra
(Licorice Root)

Licorice root is the most well-known herb for adrenal support. It has been used for centuries in Asia, and is found in almost all patented Chinese herbal formulations. Licorice has a compound in it called glycyrrhizin, which is structurally similar to cortisol, and which can bind with cortisol receptors. Thus, it can give your adrenal glands a bit of a break as your body thinks it has enough cortisol because of the glycyrrhizin. The glycyrrhizin can also increase the half-life of cortisol, allowing it to function longer in the body. One thing to mention about licorice is that it can increase blood pressure, so people with high blood pressure should avoid it.

Licorice Root (Deglycyrrhizinated Standardized Extract)	500 mg, twice daily

Step 5: Homeopathic Remedies

There are a variety of homeopathic remedies that people with low cortisol could benefit from. Please see my recommended homeopathic remedies in the Appendix.

Step 6: Hormone Replacement Support

Bioidentical Cortisol

When people are so worn down that they are unable to function in their daily life, they may require an initial round of hydrocortisone. Hydrocortisone has the exact same structure as cortisol in our bodies, so it can bind to the same receptors to trigger the same response. By supplying exogenous cortisol, your adrenal glands can take a break and focus on restoring their function without having to constantly produce cortisol. Bioidentical cortisol should not be taken in excess of 20 mg per day in the treatment of adrenal fatigue.

Bioidentical cortisol is available in a few different forms: transdermal, oral, and sublingual (under the tongue).

Cortisol replacement is covered in more detail in the "Hormone Replacement Therapy" section in the Appendix.

BIOIDENTICAL CORTISOL REPLACEMENT	
Hydrocortisone	Compounded bioidentical cortisol available in individualized doses as transdermal creams, oral tablets, and sublingual lozenges
Cortef	Brand name for bioidentical cortisol; oral formulation available in predetermined (and often too high) dosages

Case Example: Lisa, Age 54

Symptoms:

I first met Lisa when she was extremely exhausted and run-down. It was extremely difficult for her to get up in the morning, and she didn't have energy to do anything except "just be." She rated her energy at a 3 of 10. She explained that she had to quit her job two years ago because of fatigue and a persistent inability to focus and complete tasks. She was also experiencing symptoms of PMS, with irritability and migraines. She explained she had a very difficult childhood and was currently in counseling.

Diagnosis:

Based on her symptoms and lab results, Lisa was experiencing cortisol, DHEA, and progesterone deficiencies, as well as low vitamin D levels.

Treatment:

I prescribed Lisa bioidentical cortisol, DHEA, and progesterone, along with a high-quality multivitamin, omega-3 fatty acids, an adrenal herbal combination, and vitamin D. I also recommended she continue her counseling around her childhood trauma and focus on a diet high in protein and low in gluten and wheat. I mentioned to her the importance of decreasing stress, establishing a routine, and avoiding any stimulants, such as coffee and black tea.

Results:

After just one week of following my recommendations, she said she was feeling better than she could ever remember. She found herself waking up without an alarm and even going out one night with friends. She felt alive again. This new sense of energy had lasted for about two weeks until she encountered a large stressor. After this stressor, her energy plummeted again and she got another migraine. I increased her dose of the bioidentical cortisol, DHEA, and the herbal combination to try and get her back on her feet. After a few days, she was able to pull out of the slump and again felt much better.

I checked in with her six weeks later, and she said she was feeling so much better that she wanted to start work again. I advised her to wait another few months to give her adrenals some time to recover before starting a new job, where there would undoubtedly be some initial stress. Her energy was up to an 8, her migraines significantly decreased, and she was better able to deal with stress.

CHAPTER 12

Natural Solutions for Low Thyroid: Fatigue, Weight Gain, Low Mood, and Headaches

THYROID IMBALANCES can arise from various factors. We can develop an underactive thyroid because of nutritional deficiencies, stress, autoimmunity, digestive disturbance, as well as imbalances in our other hormones, such as estrogen or cortisol.

Step 1: Diet Support

In addition to the dietary guidelines outlined in the chapter "Nutrition for Happy Hormones," people with low thyroid function benefit from a diet higher in complex carbohydrates and lower in gluten and dairy products.

Increase Complex Carbohydrates

A diet higher in complex carbohydrates appears to increase thyroid hormone production, so the addition of fruits, vegetables, and whole grains is important for people experiencing low thyroid function.

Eat Brassica Vegetables in Moderation

Brassica vegetables (kale, broccoli, cabbage, cauliflower) are extremely important for our liver detoxification pathways and the metabolism of excess hormones. However, they appear to decrease thyroid function. So, if you do eat a lot of these, I suggest cutting back or cooking them, as cooking seems to lessen their inhibitory effects on the thyroid.

Avoid Dairy and Gluten

Dairy and gluten are extremely important to avoid if your low thyroid function is because of Hashimoto's thyroiditis, an autoimmune condition that targets the thyroid gland. Both gluten and dairy products have been shown to worsen the autoimmunity involved with Hashimoto's thyroiditis.

Step 2: Lifestyle Support

Healthy lifestyle choices are vital for optimal hormone balance. Adequate sleep, minimal stress, routine, healthy eating, and exercise are all important for optimal thyroid balance.

Decrease Stress

Stress downregulates our thyroid hormone production and causes an imbalance in other hormones, such as cortisol and DHEA. Think of the areas in your life that cause you the most stress and brainstorm about what you can do to decrease this.

Exercise

Exercise is another important aspect to consider. Exercise increases your metabolism and energy and promotes weight loss.

If you have hypothyroidism, even the thought of exercising may make you feel tired, so it's important to start off slow. Walking is a great way to get your body moving without too much exertion. Start off with 15-minute walks and slowly work up. Walking is also a great way to get in some "me" time and decrease stress.

Routine

Establishing a routine is also important for thyroid health. Each day of the week, try to wake up and go to bed at the same time, and eat your meals at the same times. By establishing a regular routine, your stress response will decrease, your metabolism will balance out, and you will regain some of your energy. Routine also helps with weight maintenance.

Step 3: Nutritional Support

Many people notice an improvement in their thyroid function just by replacing deficient vitamins and minerals. Deficiencies in zinc, selenium, iodine, and vitamins C and D are often associated with low thyroid function.

Zinc

Zinc is an important cofactor for the production of thyroid hormones. It is needed for the conversion of T4 to T3, our active thyroid hormone. T3 levels have been shown to increase in response to zinc supplementation alone. Zinc is found in high concentrations in oysters, beef roast, collard greens, and sunflower and pumpkin seeds, as well as other nuts and seeds.

Zinc Picolinate	20–50 mg daily*

*Can interfere with copper absorption; take 2 mg of copper for every 20 mg of zinc

Selenium

Selenium is important in reestablishing thyroid balance by assisting in the conversion of T4 to T3. Selenium supplementation has been shown to directly increase T3 levels, while decreasing reverse T3 levels.

Selenium is found in high concentrations in Brazil nuts, halibut and salmon, Swiss chard, blackstrap molasses, and oysters.

Selenium	200 mcg daily

Iodine

Iodine is found in high concentrations in the thyroid gland. It upregulates and binds with the enzyme thyroid peroxidase to produce T4 and T3. In places where iodine deficiency is common (such as Africa, Europe, and the eastern Mediterranean), supplementing with it can make a big difference in bringing your thyroid gland back into balance.

One thing to be aware of is the supplementation of iodine in Hashimoto's disease. Since Hashimoto's disease is caused by an autoimmune attack against thyroid peroxidase, upregulating it with the addition of iodine can actually make the autoimmunity worse. For people with Hashimoto's thyroiditis, I recommend avoiding extra iodine supplementation.

Iodine is found in high concentrations in kelp, arame, cod fish, halibut, sardines, and herring.

Iodine	200 mcg daily

Vitamin D3

Vitamin D3 is of particular importance for the autoimmune thyroid condition, Hashimoto's thyroiditis. Since vitamin D plays such a large role in regulating our immune system, it can actually decrease the severity of the autoimmune attack toward our thyroid gland.

Vitamin D is important not only for our thyroid health. It is also needed to maintain our bone mass, increase our mood and energy, and decrease our risk of certain types of cancer and autoimmune diseases, as well as decrease our risk of diabetes. It is a very important vitamin, and I suggest everyone have their vitamin D3 tested to ensure adequate levels.

The main source of vitamin D is sunlight. However, nowadays, with the majority of us spending up to 80 percent of our time indoors, there is no way to get enough sun exposure for adequate vitamin D production.

Vitamin D3	2,000–5,000 IU daily, depending on serum vitamin D3 levels

Thyroid Glandulars

Porcine thyroid glandulars are greatly beneficial for restoring thyroid function. They provide high-quality thyroid tissue with many different enzymes, cofactors, and nutrients required for optimal thyroid function. Many people feel an increase in energy after starting glandulars.

Thyroid Glandular (Porcine)	100 mg, 1–2 times daily

Foundation Supplements

I believe that everyone can benefit from three foundational supplements: a high-quality multivitamin, omega-3 fatty acids, and vitamin D. A high-quality multivitamin should have many of the abovementioned vitamins and minerals in adequate amounts. I have thoroughly discussed the benefits of these supplements in the chapter "Nutrition for Happy Hormones," as I think they should be part of your daily diet.

Step 4: Herbal Support

Withania somnifera
(Ashwagandha)

Ashwagandha contains phytonutrients that lead to increased production of both T4 and T3. It also acts as a powerful adrenal adaptogen by supporting our adrenal glands and modulating our stress response. If there is an accompanying adrenal and cortisol imbalance, this herb is strongly indicated as part of the thyroid-balancing program.

Ashwagandha (Dried Root)	600 mg, twice daily

Step 5: Homeopathic Remedies

There are a variety of homeopathic remedies that people with a low thyroid could benefit from. Please see my recommended homeopathic remedies in the Appendix.

Step 6: Hormone Replacement Support

Hormones are regularly prescribed for hypothyroidism. The most common prescriptions include cytomel, levothyroxine, synthroid, Armour® Thyroid, and Nature-Throid®. These hormones are beneficial in particular cases in which nutritional supplementation is inadequate for thyroid gland restoration.

Thyroid replacement is covered in more detail in the "Hormone Replacement Therapy" section in the Appendix.

THYROID HORMONE REPLACEMENT	
Levothyroxine	Synthetic thyroxine (T4)
Synthroid	Synthetic thyroxine (T4)
Nature-Throid®	Brand name for desiccated thyroid gland; it contains T3 and T4 hormones
Armour® Thyroid	Brand name for desiccated thyroid gland; it contains T3 and T4 hormones
Cytomel	Trade name for triiodothyronine (T3)

Case Example: Sarah, Age 44

Symptoms:

When I first met Sarah, she was experiencing the typical symptoms of hypothyroidism: weight gain, fatigue, and chronic headaches. She said that getting out of bed in the morning was incredibly difficult for her and that, when she got home at the end of the day, it took everything she had just to make dinner. Sarah rated her average energy as 4 of 10. Her husband was concerned that there could be something more serious going on with her health because of her constant fatigue and headaches.

Diagnosis:

Lab testing confirmed that Sarah was experiencing symptoms of low thyroid function. Her TSH was at 5.1 mIU/L, and her T3 and T4 levels were on the low end of normal.

Treatment:

I started Sarah on a high-quality multivitamin supplying optimal amounts of zinc, selenium, and iodine, as well as omega 3s, ashwagandha, and Nature-Throid® (desiccated thyroid gland that contains both T3 and T4 hormones). I also advised her to avoid gluten and dairy products.

Results:

After three weeks, Sarah was feeling more energy than she could ever remember. Her headaches disappeared and she lost seven pounds. She responded very well to this treatment program, and six months later, she was still doing great, with no recurrence of the chronic headaches, except when she didn't get enough sleep or drink enough water. Her energy level increased to 8 of 10.

CHAPTER 13

Natural Solutions for DHEA Deficiency: Poor Concentration, Abdominal Fat, and Low Libido

DEHYDROEPIANDROSTERONE (DHEA), like testosterone, is a building hormone. It promotes energy, libido, and bone strength and helps our body heal from injury. It also helps us cope with stress and increases our energy and mood.

DHEA imbalances most often show up as deficiencies; however, some conditions, such as PCOS, can predispose us to high DHEA levels as well.

DHEA levels naturally start declining in our early thirties, but, like testosterone, symptoms usually do not appear right away. As the levels of DHEA and testosterone decline with age, we are at a greater risk of age-related illnesses. This correlation is so strong that declining DHEA and testosterone levels are better markers for tracking the degenerative aging process than any other biological markers. Since DHEA is primarily produced by the adrenal glands, its production and release are greatly influenced by stress. Because of this, I often see DHEA deficiency alongside adrenal fatigue and cortisol deficiency.

Symptoms of decreasing DHEA concentrations include loss of muscle tone, difficulty concentrating, increased abdominal fat, and decreased libido.

Step 1: Diet Support

In addition to the dietary guidelines outlined in the chapter "Nutrition for Happy Hormones," people with low DHEA benefit from a diet high in protein and low in starch and sugar. Caffeine and alcohol should also be avoided.

Increase Protein

A higher protein diet, particularly of animal proteins, has been shown to increase DHEA levels. One thing to keep in mind if increasing dietary animal protein is to eat as clean as possible. This means organic, grass-fed, hormone-free, and antibiotic-free animal meats. Eating a higher protein/lower carbohydrate diet will also help balance out blood-sugar levels and promote fat loss. Try to incorporate protein with every meal.

Decrease Caffeine and Other Stimulants

Caffeine and other stimulants trigger the stress response in our bodies, so if you are already having a hard-enough time dealing with your everyday stress, these will only add more fuel to the fire. You need to focus on decreasing stress from all sources: physical, mental/emotional, and dietary.

Decrease Sugar

With every hormonal imbalance, I mention the importance of decreasing sugar. A low sugar diet is crucial for health. Increased sugar leads to blood-sugar imbalances, such as diabetes and insulin resistance, low energy, immune suppression, and an increased risk of cancer, as well as intestinal problems, behavioral disorders, and obesity, one of the leading causes of death in the United States. It is vital to decrease sugar as much as possible.

Step 2: Lifestyle Support

Healthy lifestyle choices are crucial for optimal hormone balance. Adequate sleep, exercise, and minimal stress are all important for optimizing adrenal function and DHEA levels.

Decrease Stress

Stress depletes our DHEA levels at a faster rate than normal, so it is important to find ways in which you can decrease stress. When your adrenal glands are stressed, they initially produce higher levels of all adrenal hormones, but over time, they become less sensitive to this stress and no longer produce adequate amounts (known as adrenal fatigue). Think of the areas in your life that cause you the most stress and brainstorm what you can do to decrease this. It may be looking for a new job, slowing down on nonpersonal and work commitments, or spending more time doing things you enjoy and less time doing things you don't. Meditation is also a great way to decrease stress, and I recommend it for everyone with a DHEA deficiency.

Exercise

Exercise is very healthy for us, but it is also a form of physical stress, and if your DHEA levels are low because of concomitant adrenal fatigue, you are already having a hard-enough time dealing with daily stressors. I recommend you do exercise, but keep it to the lighter exercises, such as yoga, pilates, walking, and light weight lifting.

If your lower DHEA levels are associated more with the aging process than adrenal fatigue, it is important to include weight-bearing and strength-building exercises. These types of exercise lead to increased DHEA and testosterone levels.

Routine

Establishing a routine is important for overall hormonal balance. Each day of the week, try to wake up and go to bed at the same time, and eat your meals at the same times. By establishing a regular routine, your stress response will decrease, your metabolism will balance out, and you will feel an increase in energy and mood.

Step 3: Nutritional Support

Many of the same supplements recommended for adrenal fatigue and cortisol deficiency are also useful for increasing DHEA levels. These include adrenal glandulars, vitamin C, and vitamin E.

Adrenal Glandulars and Extracts

Adrenal glandulars are adrenal supplements made up of actual adrenal gland tissue, usually from porcine or bovine sources. They provide your adrenal glands with the raw materials required to replenish and nourish themselves so they can produce adequate levels of DHEA and cortisol.

Adrenal Cortex Extracts	250 mg, 2–3 times daily

Vitamin C

Vitamin C is critical for adrenal gland function and recovery. It is a necessary cofactor for the adrenal cascade (the production of adrenal hormones from cholesterol in the adrenal glands). Without vitamin C, your adrenal glands would be unable to keep up with the hormonal demand, resulting in lower levels of cortisol and DHEA. Vitamin C also acts as a strong antioxidant and immune booster in our bodies. If you have lower levels of cortisol and DHEA and are prone to the common cold, vitamin C is definitely a supplement for you. Vitamin C can be found in high concentrations in acerola berries, guava, red chili peppers, green and sweet bell peppers, grapefruit, watermelon, kiwi, Brussels sprouts, cauliflower, and broccoli.

Vitamin C	1,000 mg, 2–3 times daily

Vitamin E

Vitamin E, like vitamin C, plays an important role in the production of adrenal hormones. It is found in the highest concentrations in the pituitary and adrenal glands and must be present in adequate amounts in order for your adrenal glands to produce optimal levels of both DHEA and cortisol. Along with its role in the production of adrenal hormones, vitamin E is also a strong antioxidant and nerve and muscle protectant. Vitamin E is found in high concentrations in almonds, hazelnuts, sunflower seeds, pecans, flaxseed oil, sunflower and safflower oil, sweet potatoes, and tempeh.

Vitamin E **(Mixed Tocopherols)**	800 IU daily

Vitamin B5

Vitamin B5 is necessary for optimal adrenal function during times of stress. It is so essential for the synthesis of adrenal hormones that, if there is a deficiency, your adrenal glands can actually shrink in size.

High concentrations of vitamin B5 can be found in chicken and beef liver, dark poultry meat, brewer's yeast, beef, eggs, and brown rice.

Vitamin B5	500 mg, twice daily

Magnesium

Magnesium, like vitamins C, E, and B5, is essential for optimally functioning adrenal glands. It is needed for the production of certain enzymes necessary for the adrenal cascade. Without it, the production of adrenal hormones, such as DHEA, would be significantly lower. Food sources of magnesium include brown rice, beans, nuts and seeds, kelp, Swiss chard, and buckwheat.

Magnesium **(Elemental or Citrate)**	400 mg daily

Foundation Supplements

I believe that everyone can benefit from three foundational supplements: a high-quality multivitamin, omega-3 fatty acids, and vitamin D. A high-quality multivitamin should have the above mentioned vitamins and minerals in adequate amounts. I've thoroughly discussed the benefits of these supplements in the chapter "Nutrition for Happy Hormones," as I think they should be part of your daily diet.

Step 4: Herbal Support

Withania somnifera
(Ashwagandha)

Ashwagandha is an extremely important herb for adrenal imbalances. It is considered an adrenal adaptogen, meaning it can bring adrenal function back into normal ranges. If your DHEA levels are too low, ashwagandha will actually work to promote adrenal hormone production, thereby bringing DHEA levels back into normal range. Besides acting as an adrenal adaptogen, ashwagandha also increases energy, strength, endurance, and libido and decreases inflammation. It is particularly useful in inflammatory conditions, such as rheumatoid arthritis and osteoarthritis, which are sometimes associated with low adrenal function.

Ashwagandha (Dried Root)	600 mg, twice daily

Eleutherococcus senticosus
(Siberian Ginseng)

Siberian ginseng, like ashwagandha, is an adrenal adaptogen. It improves mental concentration, sustains energy levels and endurance, and decreases irritability. It often has a very positive effect on mood. Siberian ginseng is also considered to be an immune-modulating herb, meaning it will strengthen the immune system so it is better able to fight off illness. People with adrenal fatigue, low cortisol, and low DHEA often end up with cold after cold because of a weakened immune system, and Siberian ginseng is a great herb to finally put an end to that cold cycle.

Siberian Ginseng (Dried Root)	800 mg, twice daily

Glycyrrhiza glabra
(Licorice Root)

Licorice root is the most well-known herb for adrenal support. It has been used for centuries in Asia and is found in almost all patented Chinese herbal formulations. Since licorice has an overall beneficial effect on the adrenal glands, it can increase the production of all adrenal hormones, including DHEA.

One thing to mention about licorice is that it can increase blood pressure in some people, so I suggest monitoring your blood pressure to make sure it doesn't rise to an unhealthy level. If you see your blood pressure rising, simply decrease your dose of licorice or discontinue it completely.

Licorice Root **(Deglycyrrhizinated** **Standardized Extract)**	500 mg, twice daily

Step 5: Homeopathic Remedies

There are a variety of homeopathic remedies that people with a DHEA deficiency could benefit from. Please see my recommended homeopathic remedies in the Appendix.

Step 6: Hormone Replacement Support

Bioidentical DHEA

DHEA supplementation often improves symptoms within two to three weeks. People notice an increase in energy and concentration, as well as better sleep and stress resistance. I have also found it to be beneficial in adrenal fatigue-related insomnia.

DHEA can be converted into testosterone, so it is important to monitor testosterone levels as well as DHEA levels when supplementing with it. DHEA can be found in many vitamin stores, but often the dose is too high, particularly for women. Five to 10 mg of DHEA are considered to be an appropriate dosage for women, whereas 25 to 100 mg is suitable for men. DHEA replacement is covered in more detail in the "Hormone Replacement Therapy" section in the Appendix.

DHEA Excess

I usually see DHEA excess only in patients taking too high a dose of exogenous DHEA or in women with polycystic ovarian syndrome. In some cases, DHEA can be increased in times of acute stress, and if this is the case, you need to decrease your stress response as much as you can. Other causes of high DHEA levels include pituitary and adrenal tumors, as well as Cushing's disease. If you are experiencing DHEA-excess symptoms and are not currently taking supplemental DHEA, I recommend you have your levels tested and evaluated by a health-care practitioner.

Case Example: Claudia, Age 41

Symptoms:
When I first met Claudia, she was experiencing fatigue, brain fog, a nonexistent libido, and difficulty getting started with work tasks. She said everything had been gradually getting worse since having had her first child one year ago. She just had no spark left.

Diagnosis:
Based on her symptoms and lab results, Claudia was experiencing adrenal fatigue with extremely low levels of DHEA

and cortisol. I also discovered she had an underlying iron and vitamin D deficiency.

Treatment:
I started Claudia on adrenal extracts, ashwagandha, and a multivitamin containing sufficient amounts of vitamins E, C, D, and B, omega 3s, and iron. I also prescribed her a bioidentical DHEA cream to help boost her DHEA levels. I mentioned to her the importance of decreasing stress, establishing a routine, and avoiding any stimulants, such as coffee and black tea.

Results:
After six weeks, Claudia's energy improved from 4 of 10 to 7 of 10. She was having an easier time focusing at work and wasn't feeling so overwhelmed with her tasks. I checked in again six weeks later, and she was still noticing improvement. The one recommendation she noticed that had made the most difference was establishing a routine. She felt more rested and in control when she stuck to her regular sleeping/ waking and eating routines.

CHAPTER 14

Natural Solutions for Testosterone Deficiency: Low Libido, Fatigue, and Increased Body Fat

TESTOSTERONE IS often thought of as a male hormone, but as we discussed in the chapter "What Are Hormones and Why Are They Important?," testosterone is also essential for women. Testosterone increases energy, builds bone and muscle mass, reduces fat, stimulates hair growth, and protects the heart and blood vessels. With optimal levels, you are better able to deal with stress and anxiety, as well as maintain an increased sense of self-confidence. Testosterone imbalances most often show up as deficiencies; however, some conditions, such as PCOS, can predispose us to high testosterone levels as well.

Testosterone naturally starts to decrease in our mid-twenties; however, symptoms do not become noticeable until about the early forties. Low testosterone levels lead to decreased energy, libido, and muscle and bone mass, a lack of self assurance, and low mood, as well as increased fat accumulation and wrinkles. Testosterone deficiency also contributes to the vaginal dryness and hot flashes experienced by postmenopausal women.

Step 1: Diet Support

In addition to the dietary guidelines outlined in the chapter "Nutrition for Happy Hormones," people with low testosterone benefit from a diet high in protein and low in starch and sugar. Caffeine and alcohol should also be avoided.

Increase Protein

A higher protein diet, particularly of animal proteins, has been shown to increase testosterone levels. One thing to keep in mind if increasing dietary animal protein is to eat as clean as possible. This means organic, grass-fed, hormone-free, and antibiotic-free animal meats. Eating a higher protein/lower carbohydrate diet will also help balance out blood-sugar levels and promote fat loss. Try to incorporate protein in every meal.

Decrease Caffeine and Other Stimulants

Caffeine and other stimulants trigger the stress response in our bodies. This stress response sways our body away from its rest state to the fight-or-flight response. When our bodies are in this state, optimal hormonal balance is not a concern.

Decrease Sugar

With every hormonal imbalance, I mention the importance of decreasing sugar. A low sugar diet is crucial for health. Increased sugar leads to blood-sugar imbalances, such as diabetes and insulin resistance, low energy, immune suppression, and an increased risk of cancer, as well as intestinal problems, behavioral disorders, and obesity, one of the leading causes of death in the United States. It is vital to decrease sugar as much as possible.

Step 2: Lifestyle Support

Healthy lifestyle choices are crucial for optimal hormone balance. Adequate sleep, minimal stress, and exercise are all important for optimizing testosterone levels.

Decrease Stress

Our bodies function best during times of rest. When our body is calm, it is able to concentrate on resetting itself back to equilibrium. This means focusing on restoring hormonal, immune, and digestive balance. It is important to find ways in which you can decrease your stress. Think of the areas in your life that cause you the most stress and brainstorm what you can do to decrease this. It may be looking for a new job, slowing down on nonpersonal and work commitments, and/or spending more time doing things you enjoy.

Moderate Exercise

Exercise is another important aspect to consider. Many studies have shown an increase in testosterone levels after exercise. This increase in testosterone leads to improved muscle mass and definition, as well as the potential for decreasing fat stores and preventing bone loss.

Sufficient Sleep

Sufficient sleep is vitally important. You need a good night's rest to function at an optimal level the next day and to respond to stress adequately. It is at night while our bodies are at rest when we are able to focus on hormone production and balance, and if we are not getting enough sleep during this time, hormones, such as thyroid-stimulating hormone, testosterone, melatonin, and insulin, will decrease.

Step 3: Nutritional Support

There are a few different testosterone-supporting vitamins, but zinc is by far one of the most important.

Zinc

Zinc deficiency is correlated with low testosterone levels and decreased sperm count and motility in men. Testosterone-deficient men supplemented with zinc show increased testosterone levels and improved sperm counts and motility. Zinc is also important because it prevents the conversion of testosterone into dihydrotestosterone (DHT), the hormone associated with male pattern baldness and prostate cancer. All people, including women, taking exogenous testosterone should ensure optimal zinc levels. Zinc is found in high concentrations in oysters, beef, turkey, dark, leafy greens, rolled oats, and pumpkin and sunflower seeds, as well as lentils and beans.

Zinc Picolinate	20–50 mg daily*

Can interfere with copper absorption; take 2 mg of copper for every 20 mg of zinc

Foundation Supplements

I believe that everyone can benefit from three foundational supplements: a high-quality multivitamin, omega-3 fatty acids, and vitamin D. A high-quality multivitamin should have the abovementioned vitamins and minerals in adequate amounts. I have thoroughly discussed the benefits of these supplements in the chapter "Nutrition for Happy Hormones," as I think they should be part of your daily diet.

Step 4: Herbal Support

Panax Ginseng
(Korean Ginseng)

Korean ginseng is an energizing herb with beneficial effects on cortisol and testosterone. It has been shown to increase the levels of both total and free testosterone, as well as cortisol. Korean ginseng leads to improved male fertility and sperm count and an increased ability to deal with acute stress. It also promotes an overall improvement in energy, libido, and endurance.

Korean Ginseng	200–400 mg daily

Tribulus terrestris
(Tribulus)

Tribulus is an herb with known androgen effects. It has been used for infertility for hundreds of years with much success. Tribulus contains phytochemicals called steroidal saponins, which have been shown to increase testosterone levels. It is thought that these saponins contribute to increased testosterone levels by inducing luteinizing hormone in the body. This is a great herb for both men and women experiencing low testosterone and/or infertility.

Tribulus **(Standardized Extract)**	200–400 mg daily

Serenoa repens
(Saw Palmetto)

Saw palmetto is considered to be a male tonic, as it generally supports the male reproductive and urinary systems. Saw palmetto doesn't directly increase testosterone levels, but instead prevents the conversion of testosterone to dihydro-testosterone (DHT), the hormone known to promote the growth of the prostate gland. DHT is implicated in benign prostate hyperplasia and prostate cancer. Saw palmetto combined with zinc significantly decreases this conversion and is beneficial for anyone (men and women) taking exog-enous testosterone, as well as for men with an increased risk of prostate cancer.

Saw Palmetto (Berry) Extract	320 mg daily

Step 5: Homeopathic Remedies

There are a variety of homeopathic remedies that people with testosterone deficiency could benefit from. Please see my recommended homeopathic remedies in the Appendix.

Step 6: Hormone Replacement Support

Bioidentical Testosterone

Many men and women are prescribed bioidentical testosterone during menopause and andropause. Men are prescribed much higher doses than women, with women using about 1/10 of the dose for men. It is important to be aware of testosterone-excess symptoms when taking bioidentical testosterone, as those symptoms indicate too high of a dose. Excess body odor, greasy hair, increased acne, and/or aggression are signs of excess testosterone.

Bioidentical testosterone is available in a few different forms: transdermal gels, oral tablets, sublingual troches, and injections. It is best to avoid oral formulations of testosterone, as the majority of it will be excreted in the urine. Testosterone replacement is covered in more detail in the "Hormone Replacement Therapy" section in the Appendix.

BIOIDENTICAL TESTOSTERONE REPLACEMENT	
Testosterone	Compounded bioidentical testosterone available in individualized doses as transdermal gels and patches, oral tablets, sublingual troches, and injections
AndroGel®	Brand name for bioidentical testosterone gel

Bioidentical DHEA

DHEA can be converted into testosterone, so, in some cases, DHEA is prescribed with the anticipation that it will increase testosterone levels. I have seen this work quite well for women, but for some reason, DHEA doesn't lead to increased testosterone concentrations in men.

DHEA is considered an over-the-counter medicine in the United States and can be bought in many vitamin stores. However, the dose found in the vitamin-store DHEA supplements is usually too high, particularly for women. Five to 10 mg of DHEA is considered an appropriate dose for women, whereas 25 to 100 mg is suitable for men. DHEA replacement is covered in more detail in the "Hormone Replacement Therapy" section in the Appendix.

Testosterone Excess

I typically see testosterone excess only in patients taking too high a dose of exogenous testosterone or in women with polycystic ovarian syndrome (PCOS). Other causes of high testosterone levels include pituitary and adrenal tumors or tumors and cysts of the testes and ovaries. If you are experiencing testosterone-excess symptoms and are not currently taking exogenous testosterone, I recommend you have your levels tested and evaluated by a health-care practitioner.

Case Example: Julie, Age 40

Symptoms:
Julie came to my practice specifically seeking bioidentical hormone replacement therapy. She explained that she worked as a personal trainer and had always lived a very healthy, active life. However, during the last two years, no matter what she did, she was not seeing any results from diet and exercise. Her muscle definition was disappearing and being replaced by fat, even though she was active with her clients every day. She thought she had low testosterone levels. Julie was also noticing that her sleep was becoming disturbed and not as restful. She was following a diet similar to the paleo diet, with decreased grains and increased animal protein and vegetables.

Diagnosis:
Based on Julie's symptoms and lab results, we discovered she indeed had low testosterone, along with a progesterone deficiency.

Treatment:
I started Julie on a higher protein diet accompanied by an amino acid formula, a high-quality multivitamin, omega-3s, *Vitex agnus-castus* (chaste-tree berry), and low dose, bioidentical testosterone and progesterone (oral progesterone to help with sleep). I also advised her to increase weight-bearing exercises.

Results:

After six weeks, Julie said her sleep and energy had improved, and she hadn't gained any weight. I retested her testosterone and progesterone levels, and they had come into the optimal range.

I checked in with Julie another six weeks later, and she said her sleep and energy levels were still improved and she was beginning to notice an improvement in her muscle definition. Her muscles didn't feel as flabby as they used to.

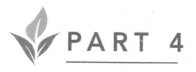

PART 4

Putting It All Together

CHAPTER 15

Getting Started with
Happy Hormones

THIS CHAPTER is all about helping you get started on
your path to happy hormones. In the previous chapters,
you learned how diet and lifestyle affect hormonal imbalance, and you also discovered what hormonal imbalances
may be affecting you and what treatment protocol would
work best for those imbalances. All this new knowledge may
feel overwhelming, and you may not know where to begin,
so to help you out, I have written this getting-started guide.

It is important to start with an outline:

1. Get organized.
2. Get started on diet and lifestyle suggestions described in
    the previous chapters.

3. Begin with the foundation supplements: a high-quality multivitamin, omega-3 fatty acids, and vitamin D.

4. Clean up your environment and personal hygiene products to decrease your exposure to harmful endocrine disruptors.

5. Book an appointment with a naturopathic doctor who is knowledgeable in hormone balancing and bioidentical hormone replacement therapy. Explain your questionnaire results and symptoms and suggest the testing you would like to have done.

6. Have lab tests done to check your nutrient status and hormone levels. If your doctor is not on board with testing your hormones, refer to the Appendix for a list of labs offering home testing.

7. Begin with your hormone-specific Happy Hormones treatment program.

8. Regularly repeat lab testing and reflect on your symptoms to monitor your improvement.

Get Organized

Reread the parts of this book that were the most meaningful for you, and then write out your plan, time line, and goals. By writing these things down, you will be more likely to move forward and achieve your end goal of balanced hormones, increased energy, decreased PMS, or whatever else it may be. I suggest posting this plan in an obvious place where you will see it every day, such as on the refrigerator, near your work desk, or on your nightstand.

As part of getting organized, I also suggest making some time for yourself. By allowing yourself this "me time," you can nourish your mind and spirit. Reserve some time to do whatever makes you feel happy and alive, whether it is going for a walk in nature, getting together with your friends, or hitting the gym.

Begin Some of the Lifestyle Suggestions

Decreasing stress, getting adequate sleep, establishing a routine, and exercising regularly are the most important lifestyle contributors to happy hormones.

Decrease Stress

Think of the areas in your life that cause you the most stress and brainstorm what you can do to decrease this. Sometimes it means slowing down on personal and work commitments, learning how to ask for help, saying no to unnecessary activities and unrealistic requests, or taking up meditation or yoga. Take some time to think about this and do what you can to decrease stress in your life.

Get Sleep

Adequate sleep is something we all need in order to function at our best. If you are not getting enough sleep, your body and mind are not running at their full capacity, which hinders your response to stress. If you are having difficulty with insomnia, seek out a naturopathic doctor to help you restore your natural sleep cycle so you can get a restful night's sleep.

Establish a Routine

Our bodies love routine. The best way to establish routine is to go to bed and wake up at the same times every day and to eat at specific times during the day. This doesn't have to be at precisely the same time every day, but if you could keep it within 30 minutes, that is best. After doing this for a couple of weeks, you will start to notice that you get hungry at the same times every day, you will start yawning at a particular time before bed, and you will even wake up without an alarm clock. You will also notice a more consistent energy level and mood.

Exercise

Exercise is extremely important for health, but keep in mind that frequent and intense exercise can contribute to hormonal imbalances and low energy. If you haven't exercised for a long time, I suggest working yourself up slowly by listening to your body and knowing when you've reached your limit. Just walking for 30 minutes per day has shown significant results in decreasing the risk of cardiovascular disease, diabetes, and many different cancers.

If stress is a constant element in your life, it may be beneficial to participate in some meditation and yoga classes, as both of these types of exercise are incredibly effective at decreasing stress. For those of you going through menopause or andropause, always include weight-bearing exercise in your fitness program to help maintain optimal bone and muscle mass.

Clean Up Your Diet

Diet affects not only hormonal health, but also cardiovascular, immune, and metabolic health. Focus on a diet high in vegetables, healthy fats and oils, and lean protein and low in packaged, processed sugary foods. From this point on, try to avoid buying anything that comes already prepared in a package or box. If it contains high fructose corn syrup, leave it on the shelf! An easy way to get started with these changes is to combine the nutrition program outlined in the chapter "Nutrition for Happy Hormones" with the recipe collection located in the Appendix. You can also access extra recipes on my website, www.dr-kristy.com.

Begin with Foundation Supplements

Get started on the Happy Hormones foundation supplements: a high-quality multivitamin, omega-3s, and vitamin D. A high-quality multivitamin will supply the necessary cofactors for liver detoxification and hormone and energy production. Omega-3s are essential for hormone synthesis, while also maintaining healthy nerves and cell membranes and decreasing our risk of inflammatory disorders, cardiovascular disease, and diabetes. Vitamin D is vital not only for optimal hormone function; it also acts as a powerful antioxidant and cancer preventative, increases mood, and helps maintain bone mass. These three supplements are the foundations of the nutritional supplement program. Visit www.dr-kristy.com for more information on these supplements.

Clean Up Your Environment

To decrease your exposure to endocrine disruptors, I suggest replacing conventional cleaning supplies with natural cleaners, avoiding plastics, drinking filtered water, and buying an air purifier for your home.

Conventional cleaning supplies contain many chemicals harmful to our health. Some contain known carcinogens (cancer-causing substances), while others contain chemicals that act as endocrine disruptors in our bodies. Check out the Environmental Working Group (www.ewg.org) for a list of clean, toxin-free cleaners.

As we learned in previous chapters, plastics contain chemicals that mimic estrogen in our bodies, potentially leading to an estrogen-excess imbalance. I strongly suggest you avoid heating and storing your food or drinks in plastic containers and that you replace your plastic water bottles with glass or stainless-steel bottles. I also recommend that, instead of drinking bottled water, you switch to filtered tap water. There are a few different types of filters for home use, including reverse osmosis systems, activated carbon, sediment, and kinetic degradation fluxion filters.

Another thing to keep in mind is your air quality at home and work. We spend about 80 percent of our time indoors, so it is important to ensure we are not breathing in too many harmful chemicals. Air fresheners, carpet, paint, perfumes, and furniture all release harmful chemicals into the air we breathe. By using a HEPA (high efficiency particulate air) filter, a large majority of these toxins are filtered out, allowing you to breathe in cleaner, healthier air.

Book an Appointment with a Naturopathic Doctor Knowledgeable in Hormone Balancing

It is important to work with a health-care practitioner during your hormonal-balancing program. They can work with you to monitor your symptoms and hormone levels and can prescribe bioidentical hormones if necessary. I know we all like to try treating ourselves at first, and this is fine in the lifestyle and diet arena, but to ensure maximal improvement and success, it is best to work with a doctor knowledgeable in nutritional supplementation and bioidentical hormone replacement therapy.

When you go in for your initial visit, bring in your questionnaire and a list of the lab tests you would like to have done. It is important you find a doctor who is willing to listen to your concerns and work with you to balance your hormones in a safe, natural way.

Lab Testing

Review the recommended lab tests found in the hormone diagnosis chapters to help you determine which tests may be best suited for you. If you would like to order the tests yourself, check out the Appendix for a list of labs offering nondoctor-ordered hormone tests.

Begin the Hormonal-Balancing Program Specific to You

Work with your new naturopathic doctor, who is knowledgeable in hormonal balancing, to get started on your comprehensive hormonal-balancing program. Remember that it is best to start with the diet and lifestyle recommendations before adding in some of the suggested nutritional supplements, herbs, homeopathics, and hormone replacement therapy. Also keep in mind that our hormones all influence each other and that, more often than not, a few different hormones will have to be balanced at the same time.

Repeat Lab Tests

If you and your doctor decide that hormone replacement therapy is an option for you, remember to have follow-up lab testing four to six weeks after starting the therapy, and then every three months for the first year to ensure appropriate dosing and optimal results. Also, keep in mind that achieving hormonal balance is a comprehensive process and will not happen overnight. It will take effort and commitment, but I promise it will be worth it in the end. I recommend dedicating a full three months to this Happy Hormones program to achieve optimal results.

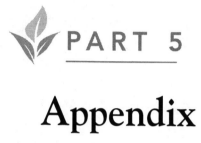

PART 5

Appendix

Hormone Replacement Therapy

ORMONE REPLACEMENT therapy was traditionally used to relieve symptoms associated with menopause, such as osteoporosis, hot flashes, insomnia, and vaginal dryness. Nowadays it is also being used in all stages of life if there is indeed a hormonal deficiency that needs extra support. Hormone replacement therapy can be particularly useful in PMS, hypothyroidism, adrenal fatigue, and for the prevention of miscarriages. Additionally, it is also being used in a preventative sense to slow the aging process and prevent the conditions and symptoms associated with aging.

As we already know, hormones protect our cardiovascular system, boost brain function, maintain bone and muscle mass, and fight off illness, infections, and inflammation. By replacing suboptimal levels of hormones, you decrease your risk of bone loss, infections, and chronic diseases, such as diabetes, arthritis, and cardiovascular disease. Having balanced hormones helps you age as healthy and energetically as possible.

One thing to remember about hormone therapy is that every person is different and needs to be treated as such. One of your friends may be receiving estrogen and testosterone replacement, but that doesn't mean you also need those, even if your symptoms are the same. For example, your symptoms of insomnia may be coming from a lack of progesterone, while your friend may have a cortisol imbalance.

There are many benefits to hormone replacement therapy, but remember that, like with many medicines, there can be risks involved. Be sure that you are taking the hormones in the safest manner possible and that your hormone levels are being monitored by a health professional knowledgeable in bioidentical hormone replacement therapy (BHRT). In this chapter, I hope to arm you with the necessary information so you can choose the safest treatment option specifically for you.

Synthetic versus Bioidentical Hormones

The naming of bioidentical and synthetic hormones can be a bit confusing, since both the bioidentical and synthetic hormones are synthesized from natural sources. The primary difference between the two is that bioidentical hormones have the exact same molecular makeup and structure as our own hormones and synthetic do not. A better name for synthetic hormones might be nonbioidentical, but for simplicity sake, we will continue referring to them as synthetic.

Bioidentical hormones have more benefits and less risks in comparison to synthetic hormones. Because bioidentical hormones have the same structure as our human hormones, they bind with the same receptors and elicit the same actions as human hormones. Synthetic hormones, on the other hand, do not bind completely with our body's receptors, resulting in an altered response and possible side effects. This can be compared to a key-and-lock model. Bioidentical hormones act as the key, fitting precisely with our cell receptors and fully opening the lock. When synthetic hormones try binding with our cell receptors, they do not quite fit and the lock doesn't fully open. This semi-opened lock will elicit a different response compared to the fully open lock seen with bioidentical hormones.

Another benefit of bioidentical versus synthetic hormones is that bioidenticals can be compounded for each individual, ensuring that you get an appropriate dose for your specific hormone levels, symptoms, and health status. Bioidentical hormones are also available in many different formulations: oral, transdermal, sublingual, and injectable. Synthetic hormones, on the other hand, come in preset doses, which are usually too high and are most often formulated as oral tablets or pills. Hormones taken orally must be processed through the liver before being absorbed into our blood stream, and when these hormones pass through the liver, (in particular estrogen), harmful by-products, such as clotting factors, binding proteins, and pro-inflammatory hormones, are formed. These by-products increase the risk of blood clots, heart disease, and strokes, as well as weight gain, sexual dysfunction, headaches, and elevations in blood pressure, triglycerides, and cholesterol.

This combination of high dosages, nonidentical molecular structure, and oral formulations are the primary reasons synthetic hormones have so many side effects. It is estimated that about half of women stop their synthetic hormones due to these side effects.

The National Heart, Lung, and Blood Institute's Women's Health Initiative, a 15-year-long study launched in 1991, examined the use of synthetic estrogen and synthetic progesterone in 161,000 postmenopausal women. The results were so astounding that the study had to be stopped early because of side effects. Women taking these synthetic hormones showed an increased risk of breast and ovarian cancers, heart disease, and strokes. The cause of these side effects was a bit blurry, but researchers suspect it was a combination of the use of oral estrogens, too high of doses, and the fact that both the estrogen and progesterone were synthetic and didn't structurally match our human equivalent. This study is a primary reason the use of hormone replacement therapy is considered risky and unsafe. The good news is that bioidentical hormones, when prescribed appropriately, possess none of these features and are not only extremely effective at low doses, but are also significantly safer than synthetic hormones. Bioidentical hormones are also associated with lower risks of breast cancer and cardiovascular disease and are more efficacious than their synthetic counterparts.

	Bioidentical Hormones	Synthetic Hormones
Identical to human hormones	Yes	No
Allow for individual dosing	Yes	No
Significantly fewer side effects	Yes	No

Synthetic Estrogen

Synthetic estrogens are a group of patented estrogen formulations that have a different molecular makeup and structure from our human estrogen. There are a few different types, but the most commonly prescribed synthetic estrogen and the one involved in the Women's Health Initiative study is called Premarin®. Premarin is a mixture of conjugated equine (horse) estrogens with estrone. There are three important facts to consider with Premarin:

Estrone is already present in high levels during menopause and is something you don't need in excess. Estrone and its metabolites are associated with increased growth of breast and uterine tissue. Humans are not designed to break down horse estrogen; we are designed to metabolize our own human estrogens. The horse estrogen can stay in the body for a longer period of time, leading to potential side effects.

Synthetic hormones are formulated as oral tablets. When estrogen is taken orally, it is metabolized by the liver, resulting in harmful by-products, such as clotting factors, binding proteins, and pro-inflammatory molecules.

While synthetic estrogens have these side effects, bio-identical estrogens do not. When prescribed for the individual in low dosages and appropriately monitored with lab testing, bioidentical hormones have significantly fewer side effects.

Synthetic (Non-Bioidentical) Estrogen Formulations	
Premarin®	Femtrace®
Cenestin®	Menest®
Enjuvia®	Ortho-Est®
Bioidentical Estrogen Formulations	
Estradiol	Estrace®
Estriol	Gynodiol®
Bi-estrogen	Vivelle-Dot®
Tri-estrogen	

Synthetic Progesterone

Synthetic progesterone is often classified as progestin. Like estrogen, synthetic progesterone has a different molecular makeup and does not fit the same receptor sites as our human progesterone. In the Women's Health Initiative study, the synthetic progesterone, Provera®, was associated with increased blood clotting, weight gain, and an increased risk of breast cancer. It has been shown to increase C-reactive protein (a marker of inflammation) and constrict our blood vessels, and is harmful during pregnancy. It is no wonder that hormone replacement therapy has had such a bad reputation. The good news is that, like bioidentical estrogen, bioidentical progesterone is considerably safer than synthetic progesterone. In some instances, it actually has the opposite effect as the synthetic progestins.

Synthetic (Non-Bioidentical) Progesterone Formulations	
Provera®	Curretab®
Cycrin®	Aygestin®
Amen®	
Bioidentical Progesterone Formulations	
Progesterone	Prometrium®

	Bioidentical Progesterone	Synthetic Progesterone (Progestin)
Heart attack risk	Decreased	Increased
Stroke risk	Decreased	Increased
Breast cancer risk	Decreased	Increased
Vaginal bleeding	Decreased	Increased

Bioidentical Hormone Benefits

Both synthetic and bioidentical hormones can have a positive effect on the symptoms of menopause and andropause. However, bioidentical hormones, when prescribed appropriately, come with less risk. They have been shown to:

- Reduce hot flashes, night sweats, and vaginal dryness and thinning

- Prevent osteoporosis

- Maintain greater muscle mass and strength

- Protect against heart attacks and strokes

- Improve blood-cholesterol levels

- Reduce the risks of uterine and breast cancers

- Reduce the risk of depression

- Improve sleep, mood, concentration, and memory

- Prevent senility and Alzheimer's disease

- Enhance libido/sex drive

How to Use Bioidentical Hormones

Research has shown that bioidentical hormones have significantly less risks than synthetic hormones when they are prescribed appropriately: transdermal (in most cases) in low doses and fitted for the individual.

Bioidentical hormones can be prescribed in various forms, including sublingual, oral, and transdermal, as creams, gels, and patches. We have already learned that oral formulations can lead to unwanted by-products when they are metabolized in the liver. One such unwanted metabolite produced from oral estrogen is called estrone sulfate, which has been associated with an increased risk of endometrial and breast cancer. Transdermal absorption allows the hormones to bypass the liver, thus preventing the harmful unwanted liver metabolites and closely mimicking the rate and rhythm that our bodies naturally produce and release hormones.

Skin creams and gels are what I most often prescribe because they allow for individual dosing, prolonged absorption, and the avoidance of the liver pathways. However, with creams and gels, compliance can sometimes be an issue. Some people find it takes more effort and time to apply transdermal creams than to swallow a pill. Another aspect to consider with transdermal application is the possibility of hormone buildup and storage. Some hormones, such as estrogen, are stored in our fat cells, and in some women, transdermal applications can actually promote this storage. This is just another reason why it is important to have follow-up lab testing with a health-care practitioner knowledgeable in hormone replacement therapy. Transdermal patches are also an option as they allow for high compliancy. The disadvantage is that they come in preset dosages and ratios, so they are difficult to adjust for each individual.

Bioidentical hormones are available for many different hormones, including estrogen, progesterone, DHEA, testosterone, cortisol, pregnenolone, and growth hormone. When using bioidentical hormones, it is important to remember that all of the hormones work together and influence each other. Because of this, you must take into consideration your overall hormonal balance and balance the hormones together rather than just working on one hormone.

Before starting on a program of bioidentical hormone replacement therapy, it is necessary to have your hormone levels tested to establish a baseline from which your levels and dose can be monitored and compared. It is important to discuss your individual symptoms, risks, and health goals with a knowledgeable health-care practitioner to ensure bioidentical hormone replacement is an appropriate line of treatment for you. There is risk with everything, but if dosed appropriately and monitored properly, bioidentical hormones are an excellent option to restore deficient hormones.

Bioidentical Estrogen

Bioidentical estrogen is most often prescribed in postmenopausal women to relieve symptoms of hot flashes, night sweats, and memory loss, as well as to prevent osteoporosis. Some premenopausal women may also need extra estrogen support if, for example, they are having irregular menstrual cycles or a complete absence of their menstrual period. Most women who begin bioidentical estrogen replacement therapy feel almost immediate relief from their hot flashes, night sweats, and irritability. It is important, however, to watch for signs of excess dosing, such as heavy periods, tender and swollen breasts, and/or irritability when taking estrogen replacement. If you have these symptoms, it means your dose is too high and needs to be decreased. In addition, women with a personal or family history of estrogen-associated breast or uterine cancer must be monitored closely when using bioidentical estrogen therapy, as estrogen normally increases the growth of these tissues. To help offset this effect, it is important to take bioidentical progesterone along with the estrogen. Progesterone opposes the effect estrogen has on breast and uterine tissue, thus decreasing the risk of estrogen-related breast and uterine cancer.

Formulations

Bioidentical estrogen can be prescribed in a variety of formulations and delivery methods. I strongly urge you to avoid oral formulations, as they lead to unwanted and potentially harmful by-products when metabolized by the liver. Transdermal and sublingual are considered to be the safest delivery methods for estrogen.

Formulations not only vary in the delivery form, but also in the type of estrogen. Some contain only estradiol, some a combination of estriol and estradiol, and others a combination of estriol, estradiol, and estrone. Remember that postmenopausal women usually have enough estrone, so it is often better to choose a formulation without this particular estrogen. If osteoporosis is a concern, a formulation containing estradiol is important, as estradiol is the estrogen that helps block the breakdown of bone tissue. See the table on the following page for the most common bioidentical estrogen formulations.

BIOIDENTICAL ESTROGEN FORMULAS		
Oral	Transdermal Creams and Gels	Transdermal Patches
Estradiol	Estradiol	Alora® (Estradiol)
Estriol	Estriol	Estraderm® (Estradiol)
Bi-estrogen (Estradiol and Estriol)	Bi-estrogen (Estradiol and Estriol)	Vivelle-Dot® (Estradiol)
Tri-estrogen (Estradiol, Estriol, and Estrone)	Tri-estrogen (Estradiol, Estriol, and Estrone)	Esclim® (Estradiol)
Estrace® (Estradiol)	Divigel® (Estradiol)	Menostar® (Estradiol)
Gynodiol® (Estradiol)	EstroGel® (Estradiol)	Climara® (Estradiol)
	Elestrin® (Estradiol)	

Important Things to Remember

- Bioidentical estrogen should be prescribed at the lowest effective dose and for the shortest time necessary as consistent with the treatment goals of, and risks to, the individual

- Estrogen should always be combined with bioidentical progesterone

- Never take oral estrogens
- Monitor for estrogen-excess symptoms and modify dose as needed

Bioidentical Progesterone

Bioidentical progesterone, like estrogen, is most often prescribed to relieve the symptoms of menopause. However, I also prescribe it to help regulate the menstrual cycle, decrease the risk of miscarriage, and resolve symptoms of PMS, insomnia, and anxiety. With the increasing occurrence of estrogen dominance, I am seeing more and more premenopausal symptoms with progesterone-deficiency symptoms.

It is important to cycle progesterone in premenopausal women so their menstrual cycle stays on track. Progesterone is used during the second phase of the menstrual cycle (days 14–28). Like with estrogen, it is important to monitor for symptoms of excess progesterone and adjust the dose if necessary. Increased weight gain, sleepiness, low libido, and low mood are signs of excess progesterone. As with estrogen therapy, women with a history of progesterone-related breast cancer should be monitored closely by a knowledgeable health-care practitioner.

Formulations

Progesterone is available in a variety of formulas and delivery methods. It is one hormone that can be taken orally, as it doesn't lead to the production of harmful metabolites through liver metabolism. Oral progesterone is particularly useful for women experiencing insomnia, as it decreases anxiety and promotes sleep. See the table below for the most common bioidentical progesterone formulations.

BIOIDENTICAL PROGESTERONE FORMULATIONS	
Oral	Transdermal Creams and Gels
Progesterone	Progesterone
Prometrium®	

Bioidentical Testosterone

Bioidentical testosterone is commonly prescribed for men and women experiencing symptoms of andropause and menopause respectively. The dose for men is much higher than that for women, as women naturally have significantly lower levels of testosterone. I generally prescribe bioidentical testosterone more for men than for women, as women's testosterone levels often improve with DHEA supplementation.

Men and women taking bioidentical testosterone often notice increased libido, energy, and muscle strength, as well as increased confidence and self-assurance. Testosterone may also decrease abdominal fat stores.

Formulations

Like estrogen and progesterone, bioidentical testosterone is available in different delivery methods and formulations.

It can be prescribed as sublingual pouches, injectables, oral tablets, or transdermal patches and creams. It is best to avoid oral formulations, as a large majority of oral testosterone is lost in the urine. Synthetic testosterone does exist, but should not be used, as it does not exactly mimic the effects of our human testosterone and has been linked with liver cancer.

When taking testosterone, it is important to monitor for excess symptoms, such as aggression and increased body hair and odor, as well as greasy hair and skin. If you have these symptoms, your dose should be decreased.

Another important fact to consider with testosterone replacement is testosterone's ability to be converted into estrogen and dihydrotestosterone (DHT). Some people rapidly convert testosterone into estrogen and/or dihydrotestosterone, so it is also important to monitor estrogen and dihydrotestosterone levels along with testosterone. See the table below for the most common bioidentical testosterone formulations.

BIOIDENTICAL TESTOSTERONE FORMULATIONS			
Oral	Transdermal Creams and Gels	Injectable	Transdermal Patches
Testosterone	Testosterone	Testosterone	Androderm®
	AndroGel®		
	Testim®		
	Fortesta		

Bioidentical Cortisol

In my practice, I sometimes prescribe bioidentical cortisol for those who are incredibly tired and suffering from adrenal fatigue and cortisol deficiency. In some cases, no matter how many herbs, vitamins, or extracts I give a patient, only the bioidentical cortisol will achieve results in the beginning. Of course, when considering adrenal fatigue, it's also important to decrease stress to an absolute minimum and adapt healthy sleep and eating patterns.

Bioidentical cortisol can increase concentration and mood, while decreasing foggy mind, irritability, and anxiety. When taking bioidentical cortisol, your symptoms and cortisol levels must be closely monitored by a knowledgeable health-care practitioner, as too much cortisol can lead to unwanted side effects. Excess symptoms can include a bloated face, increased abdominal fat, anxiety and stress, and/or thinning skin. Bioidentical cortisol supplementation, for the treatment of adrenal fatigue, should not exceed 20 mg per day.

It is important to mimic your body's natural release of cortisol to prevent any imbalances with your circadian rhythm. Our bodies release cortisol in higher concentrations in the morning and in lower concentrations throughout the afternoon, evening, and night.

Formulations

See the table below for the most common bioidentical cortisol formulations.

BIOIDENTICAL CORTISOL FORMULATIONS	
Oral	*Transdermal Creams and Gels*
Cortef®	Hydrocortisone

Bioidentical Dehydroepiandrosterone (DHEA)

Bioidentical DHEA is prescribed for both men and women; however, the dose for women is significantly lower than for men. Low DHEA levels are associated with menopause, andropause, smoking, stress, aging, and adrenal fatigue. In my practice, I most commonly prescribe DHEA during menopause and adrenal fatigue.

DHEA supplementation can result in increased energy, mood, libido, and concentration, as well as decreased anxiety and irritability. While taking DHEA, it is important to watch out for excess symptoms of increased facial hair, acne, and greasy hair.

Formulations

Like the other bioidentical hormones, DHEA is available in different formulations and delivery methods. It is one of the hormones that is available without a prescription, often in oral formulations. However, even though it is available over the counter, it is important to have a knowledgeable healthcare practitioner monitor your dose and progress. Sublingual and transdermal formulations are recommended over oral formulations. See the table below for the most common bioidentical DHEA formulations.

BIOIDENTICAL DHEA FORMULATIONS	
Oral	*Transdermal Creams and Gels*
DHEA	DHEA

Thyroid Hormone Support

Thyroid hormones are often prescribed for anyone experiencing hypothyroid symptoms, such as weight gain, fatigue, dry skin, and low mood. Most doctors prescribe levothyroxine (T4); however, many hypothyroid patients have trouble converting this T4 into the active hormone triiodothyronine (T3). Because of this, it is often beneficial to include small doses of T3 to ensure optimal results. When taking thyroid hormones, it is important to start with a low dose and slowly work your way up every 10 days. It is important to monitor yourself for excess symptoms, such as heart palpitations, increased pulse and sweating, talking fast, increased thirst and appetite, and over-the-top energy. If you feel these symptoms, you need to decrease your dose and have your thyroid lab values reevaluated.

Formulations

Thyroid hormones are available in a few different oral formulations. Some are derived from porcine glandulars, while others are strictly T4 and T3 preparations. There is some confusion over which of these thyroid formulas are synthetic and which are natural and/or bioidentical. The natural porcine-derived thyroid preparations contain bioidentical T4 and T3, with the addition of T1 and T2 thyroid hormones and some other nutrients necessary for optimal thyroid function. Synthetic preparations, such as synthroid and cytomel, also contain bioidentical T4 and T3, but are missing the extra benefits of T1 and T2.

I generally prefer the natural thyroid preparations, as they contain both T4 and T3, as well as other nutrients normally present in healthy thyroid glands. Even though the majority of my patients do very well with the natural preparations, some patients have trouble with the higher T3 to T4 ratio found in these formulas.

Thyroid dosing is very individual, and some people respond better to the natural porcine-derived formulations, while others respond better to the T4 or T3 only formulations. See the table on the following page for the most common thyroid hormone formulations.

THYROID HORMONE FORMULATIONS (ORAL)	
Formulation	
Armour Thyroid®	Porcine glandular containing levothyroxine (T4) and triiodothyronine (T3)
Nature-Throid®	Porcine glandular containing levothyroxine (T4) and triiodothyronine (T3)
Westhroid™	Porcine glandular containing levothyroxine (T4) and triiodothyronine (T3)
Cytomel®	Contains triiodothyronine (T3)
Liothyronine	Contains triiodothyronine (T3)
Synthroid®	Contains levothyroxine (T4)
Levothroid®	Contains levothyroxine (T4)
Levoxyl®	Contains levothyroxine (T4)
Thyrolar®	Contains fixed ratios of levothyroxine (T4) and triiodothyronine (T3)

Summary

Bioidentical hormone replacement therapy has many benefits and can significantly reduce the risk of age-related illnesses such as cardiovascular disease and cancer. Not only can it reduce the risk of illness, but it also can result in increased energy levels, mood, and libido and an overall sense of wellness. Many of my patients tell me how young they look and feel compared to their friends of the same age, and I can see it on the inside by monitoring their blood values.

But like many therapies, if bioidentical hormone replacement is not appropriately prescribed and monitored, some side effects and risks may occur. To ensure you get the optimal results and to decrease any risks, it is important to follow these guidelines:

- Copy nature

- Use the exact molecular duplicates of the human hormones in similar quantities normally found in our bodies

- Remember it is best to take estrogen and testosterone as transdermal preparations (or sublingual if poor transdermal absorption)

- Monitor hormone levels regularly

- Work with a doctor knowledgeable in bioidentical hormone replacement therapy

- Knowledgeable doctors can evaluate your hormone levels and your individual risk, as well as modify your dosages if necessary to ensure optimal results and success

- Remember all our hormones work together and, together, they must be balanced

Specialty Labs for Hormone Self-Testing

Here is a list of the specialty labs I commonly recommend and use for hormone testing. For the majority of hormone testing, I recommend blood testing, but in some cases (such as when testing adrenal function or urinary metabolites), salivary and urinary testing is also recommended.

Meridian Valley (www.meridianvalleylab.com)

Meridian Valley specializes in comprehensive, 24-hour urinary hormone and metabolite testing. They can send the collection test kits directly to your address.

ZRT Laboratory (www.zrtlab.com)

ZRT specializes in salivary hormone and blood spot tests. They offer salivary adrenal and hormone profiles, along with thyroid and vitamin D blood spot tests.

DirectLabs (www.directlabs.com)

You can order significantly discounted hormonal blood tests directly through DirectLabs. This is a great option if your physician is unwilling to order them for you. All you have to do is order the tests online, print out the requisition form, and then take that form to LabCorp (www.labcorp.com) to have your blood drawn. They notify you by e-mail when the results are in.

Life Extension® (www.lef.org)

Life Extension is a membership site offering significant savings on member lab testing. You just have to print out the requisition form and take it with you to LabCorp to have your blood drawn. Your results are sent directly to you.

Homeopathic Remedies for Happy Hormones

THE HOMEOPATHIC remedies shown on the following pages are some of the most commonly prescribed homeopathics for women experiencing hormonal imbalances. These constitutional homeopathics are very individual, and personality and behavioral traits need to be included with the physical symptoms in order to find the right remedy for each individual. Homeopathy concentrates on balancing the whole person, and in order for this to happen, both body and mind need to be considered.

I recommend working with a homeopathic or naturopathic doctor who is knowledgeable in homeopathy to help you find the right remedy for you. Adding the right homeopathic medicines to your Happy Hormones program can be extremely beneficial, allowing you to release any negative energy and emotions that may be holding you back from achieving the best results possible.

Calcarea Carbonica

This remedy is sometimes used to help relieve symptoms associated with low thyroid function. It is generally indicated for overweight, sedentary people who have a tendency to feel chilly and are often prone to lymph and circulatory problems, obesity, and constipation. In addition to its use for low thyroid function, it is also beneficial for the swelling and water retention associated with PMS.

Ignatia

This remedy is useful for hormonal imbalances that come on after grief. It is generally indicated for women who experience an absence of menstrual bleeding during grief. *Ignatia* is often beneficial for perfectionists who suffer from grief-related insomnia and feel irritable and betrayed. Women in need of *ignatia* frequently sigh to relieve some of their tension.

Lachesis

This is a great remedy for hormonal imbalances. Women in need of *lachesis* often experience an immediate improvement in PMS symptoms, such as headaches (often on the left side), swelling, and irritability, with the onset of menses (menstrual period). It is also beneficial for women experiencing hot flashes during menopause. In terms of personality, *lachesis* is generally indicated for jealous and suspicious people who have a tendency to lash out and have a fear of snakes and a dislike for tight clothing.

Lycopodium

Lycopodium is useful for people experiencing low thyroid function with accompanying gastrointestinal upset and poor digestion. It is generally indicated for people with low mood, feelings of insecurity, apprehension, and menstrual periods that occur late and last too long.

Natrum Muriaticum

Like the homeopathic remedy *ignatia*, *natrum muriaticum* also benefits women with hormonal imbalances that come on after grief or disappointed love. It can be used for irregular menstrual cycles, PMS, and menopausal symptoms. It is generally indicated for perfectionist women who repress their feelings, are unable to cry, and feel worse with consolation (at least initially). *Natrum muriaticum* works well for women who are reserved, quiet, and very proper.

Nux-vomica

This remedy is generally indicated for type-A personalities with stimulant cravings and a sensitivity to light, noise, and odors. This remedy works well for cortisol, estrogen, and progesterone imbalances. It is a typical remedy for imbalances due to excesses, whether it is an excess of food or alcohol, stress, and/or work. These excesses often result in irritability, headaches, digestive upset, and bad temper. *Nux-vomica* also benefits women experiencing irregular and short menstrual cycles accompanied by painful menstrual cramps extending to the lower back with a constant urging for a bowel movement.

Phosphorus

Phosphorus is a great remedy for women having intermittent spotting during their menstrual cycle and/or menstrual periods that are heavy and last too long. It is often suited for easygoing, effervescent women who are sympathetic, extremely friendly, independent, and prone to respiratory complaints.

Pulsatilla

Pulsatilla is a great remedy for women with a mild, gentle, and yielding disposition. *Pulsatilla* is generally indicated for hormonal imbalances resulting in amenorrhea and menstrual periods that are constantly changing. It is also useful for the irritability and emotional outbursts often associated with PMS. Women suited to *Pulsatilla* often feel better with open air, love, and consolation and are often emotionally needy.

Sepia

Sepia is indicated in a variety of hormonal imbalances when there are complaints of irritability and an indifference to others, particularly loved ones (children and spouse). *Sepia* works great for pregnancy complaints, such as morning sickness, PMS, menopause with night sweating and/or hot flashes, and painful menstrual periods accompanied by a bearing-down sensation in the pelvis. *Sepia* is also indicated for women with varicose veins, vaginal candida, and skin complaints associated with the menstrual cycle.

Staphysagria

Staphysagria is indicated for a variety of hormonal imbalances, particularly when there is a history of sexual abuse. It is generally useful for sweet but suppressed women who frequently try to please others. They often suppress their anger to the point where they are ready to explode. *Staphysagria* is also great for women prone to pelvic pain and/or genito-urinary infections, such as candida, and is quite helpful in decreasing outbursts and irritability associated with PMS.

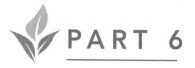

PART 6

Happy Hormones Recipe Collection

Vegetarian Omelet

Total prep and cooking time: 25 minutes

Serves 1–2

2 organic eggs
1 handful spinach
1 tomato, diced
½ small zucchini, diced
¼ cup mushrooms, chopped
Pinch salt and pepper

Whisk eggs in a small bowl, and then add to a frying pan.

Cook eggs for 2–3 minutes until the eggs begin to set on the bottom of the pan.

Gently lift the edges of the omelet with a spatula to let the uncooked part of the eggs flow toward the edges and cook.

Add the spinach, tomato, zucchini, and mushrooms.

Using a spatula, gently fold one edge of the omelet over the vegetables.

Cook for another 3 minutes.

Slide the omelet out of the skillet and onto a plate.

Cut in half and serve.

Fruit Salad with Pumpkin Seeds

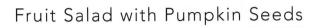

Total prep and cooking time: 10 minutes

Serves 1–2

⅓ cup fresh blueberries

⅓ cup fresh strawberries

⅓ cups fresh blackberries

¼ cup organic, gluten-free granola

2 tablespoons pumpkin seeds

Mix together in a bowl. Serve immediately.

Ginger and Walnut Oatmeal

Total prep and cooking time: 20 minutes

Serves 3

2 cups water

1 cup rolled oats

¼ cup raisins

2 teaspoons grated ginger

1 tablespoon sunflower seeds

1 tablespoon walnuts

Salt, to taste

Bring water to a boil.

Add oats, raisins, ginger, and a pinch of salt.

Reduce heat to low.

Continue cooking until water is absorbed and oats become creamy (about 7 minutes).

Add sunflower seeds and walnuts. Serve immediately.

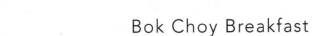

Bok Choy Breakfast

Total prep and cooking time: 25 minutes

Serves 1

BREAKFAST

4 big bok choy leaves

1 teaspoon toasted sesame oil

1 tablespoon rice vinegar

1 tablespoon tamari

½ cup cooked brown rice

Wash bok choy and chop into bite-size pieces.

Heat sesame oil in a sauté pan.

Add bok choy and stir-fry for 1 minute.

Add vinegar, tamari, and rice.

Stir gently and continue cooking (about 3 minutes) until everything is warm.

Transfer to a bowl to eat.

Roasted Tomato Basil Soup

Total prep and cooking time: 1 hour 30 minutes

Serves 6

3 pounds ripe plum tomatoes, cut in quarters

1 tablespoon high-quality olive oil

1 teaspoon sea salt

1 teaspoon freshly ground black pepper

2 yellow onions, chopped

6 cloves garlic, minced

2 tablespoons grapeseed oil

¼ teaspoon crushed red pepper flakes

1 (28 oz.) can plum tomatoes, with their juice

4 cups fresh basil leaves

1 teaspoon fresh thyme leaves

1 quart vegetable stock or water

Preheat the oven to 400°F.

Toss together the tomatoes, 1 tablespoon olive oil, salt, and pepper. Spread the tomatoes in 1 layer on a baking sheet and roast for 45 minutes.

In an 8-quart stockpot over medium heat, sauté the onions and garlic with 2 tablespoons grapeseed oil and the red pepper flakes for 10 minutes until the onions start to brown. Add the canned tomatoes, basil, thyme, and vegetable stock or water.

Add the oven-roasted tomatoes, including the liquid on the baking sheet. Bring to a boil and simmer uncovered for 40 minutes.

Taste for seasonings. Serve hot or cold.

Mulligatawny Soup

Total prep and cooking time: 1 hour 15 minutes

Serves 6

3 tablespoons grapeseed oil

1 large onion, chopped

3 stalks celery, chopped

½ teaspoon cayenne pepper

1 teaspoon turmeric

1 teaspoon coriander

1 teaspoon curry powder

2 tablespoons tamari soy sauce

6 cups water

2 medium carrots, sliced

2 large potatoes, cut into ½-inch cubes

½ cup brown rice

1 red pepper, diced

1 green pepper, diced

1 tomato, diced

1 cup cauliflower, chopped

¾ cup grated unsweetened coconut

3 teaspoons lemon juice

In a large soup pot, heat oil over medium and cook onions and celery for about 5 minutes until onions are translucent.

Add cayenne, turmeric, coriander, curry, tamari, water, carrots, potatoes, and rice. Bring to a boil, reduce heat, cover, and simmer for 20 minutes.

Add peppers, tomato, cauliflower, coconut, and lemon juice. Let simmer covered for 15–20 minutes more until vegetables and rice are tender.

Remove and blend half of the soup in a blender or food processor. Return blended soup to pot.

Serve warm.

Creamy Broccoli Soup

Total prep and cooking time: 40 minutes

Serves 4

1 medium onion, chopped

2 cloves garlic, minced

1 tablespoon grapeseed oil

5 cups vegetable broth

2 bunches broccoli, chopped

1 carrot, chopped

1 cup cooked brown rice

Sauté onion and garlic in 1 tablespoon of grapeseed oil until translucent.

In a pot, bring vegetable broth to a boil.

Add broccoli, carrot, and sautéed onion.

Reduce heat and simmer for 15 minutes.

Add brown rice and stir.

Put soup in the blender and blend until smooth.

Return soup to pot and cook for another 5 minutes. Serve warm.

Lentil Soup

Total prep and cooking time: 1 hour 10 minutes

Serves 4

½ cup red or green lentils
1 cup chopped onion
2 cloves garlic, crushed
1 stalk celery, chopped
2 carrots, chopped
2 cups shredded cabbage
2 cups vegetable broth

1 (28 oz.) can whole tomatoes, chopped
1 teaspoon salt
½ teaspoon ground black pepper
¼ teaspoon white sugar
½ teaspoon dried basil and thyme
¼ teaspoon curry powder

Place the lentils into a large pot and add water to twice the depth of the lentils. Bring to a boil, and then lower heat and let simmer for about 15 minutes.

Drain and rinse lentils; return them to the pot.

Sauté onion, garlic, celery, carrots, and cabbage for 5 minutes.

Add sautéed onion, garlic, celery, cabbage, vegetable broth, and tomatoes to the pot containing the lentils and season with salt, pepper, sugar, basil, thyme, and curry.

Cook, simmering for 1 hour. Serve warm.

Quinoa Salad

Total prep and cooking time: 30 minutes

Serves 8

2 cups cooked quinoa

2 cups fresh spinach, chopped

⅓ cup radishes, chopped

⅓ cup cucumber, chopped

⅓ cup celery, chopped

⅓ cup red onion, chopped

⅓ cup chopped red bell pepper

⅓ cup almonds, chopped

2 tablespoons olive oil

1 tablespoon balsamic vinegar

Combine all ingredients together in a big bowl.

Mix well and serve.

SALADS

SALADS

Fennel and Beet Salad

Total prep and cooking time: 50 minutes

Serves 6

4 large beets, chopped in ¼-inch pieces

2 small fennel bulbs, thinly sliced

1 bunch mint leaves, thinly sliced

3 oranges, juiced

¼ cup balsamic vinegar

3 tablespoons sunflower seeds

Boil beets in a large pot for 20–30 minutes until a fork pierces easily through the middle of each beet.

When beets are cooked, drain and rinse with cold water.

Chop the beets into ¼-inch pieces (if not already done).

Add all ingredients into a large bowl and mix well.

Sprinkle sunflower seeds on top and serve.

Chickpea and Spinach Salad

Total prep and cooking time: 1 hour

Serves 4

32 ounces cooked chickpeas (or 2 cans organic chickpeas, drained and rinsed)

1 large red onion, thinly sliced

1 large red or yellow pepper, chopped

1 cup spinach, chopped

4 tablespoons fresh cilantro, chopped

2 cloves garlic, crushed

3 tablespoons olive oil

Juice 1½ limes

Drain and rinse the canned chickpeas (if using).

Combine with onion, pepper, spinach, and cilantro.

Mix together the garlic, olive oil, and lime juice. Pour over the chickpea mixture and mix well.

Chill in the refrigerator for at least 30 minutes to allow the chickpeas to absorb the flavors. Serve chilled.

Spicy Thai Salad

Total prep and cooking time: 40 minutes

Serves 4 as side dish, 2 as main course

Salad Dressing

1 tablespoon lime juice

1 tablespoon soy sauce

1 tablespoon fish sauce (vegetarians: substitute 1 tablespoon tamari)

1 teaspoon white wine vinegar or rice vinegar

2–3 cloves fresh garlic, minced

1 fresh red chili, deseeded and minced, or ¼–½ teaspoon dried, crushed chili

1 pinch black pepper

1–2 teaspoon white sugar (to taste)

Salad

1 large English cucumber, sliced into ½-inch pieces

1 carrot, grated

1 cup whole roasted unsalted cashews

1 red bell pepper, sliced thinly

2 green onions, sliced

1 bunch fresh cilantro

2 large handfuls mixed leafy greens

First make the dressing by mixing all salad dressing ingredients together in the bowl.

Taste-test for sourness/spiciness and set aside.

Add the cucumber, grated carrot, cashews, red pepper, and green onions to a large bowl.

Pour the dressing over and toss well.

Place salad on a mixed bed of fresh cilantro and leafy greens.

Serve immediately.

Avocado and Orange Salad

Total prep and cooking time: 15 minutes

Serves 4

Salad Dressing
2 tablespoons olive oil
2 tablespoons balsamic vinegar
Pinch salt and pepper

Salad
4 large handfuls mixed salad greens
2 oranges
2 avocados
¼ cup pumpkin seeds

Combine olive oil, balsamic vinegar, salt, and pepper in a small bowl.

Place mixed salad, oranges, avocados, and pumpkin seeds in a large salad bowl.

Pour dressing over salad and serve immediately.

Black Bean and Quinoa-Filled Peppers

Total prep and cooking time: 1 hour 15 minutes

Serves 4

2 tablespoons grapeseed oil

1 medium onion, chopped finely

3 cloves garlic, crushed

2 cups mushrooms, chopped finely

1 tablespoon chili powder

1 teaspoon salt

¾ cup quinoa

1 (15 oz.) can crushed tomatoes

¼ cup water

1 (15 oz.) can black beans, drained and rinsed

3 teaspoons maple syrup

4 large red bell peppers, deseeded with tops cut off

Preheat oven to 400°F.

Heat grapeseed oil in a pan over medium heat and sauté onions 3–5 minutes until translucent and fragrant.

Add garlic and mushrooms and sauté another 5 minutes. Stir in chili powder and salt.

Add the quinoa with 1 cup of the crushed tomatoes and water.

Lower the heat and cover, simmering for 15–20 minutes until quinoa is cooked.

Add in the black beans and maple syrup and mix thoroughly.

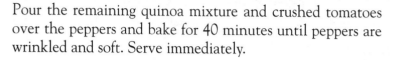

Stuff the quinoa and black bean mixture into the peppers and place into a baking dish.

Pour the remaining quinoa mixture and crushed tomatoes over the peppers and bake for 40 minutes until peppers are wrinkled and soft. Serve immediately.

VEGETARIAN MAIN COURSES

Portobello Ratatouille with Quinoa

Total prep and cooking time: 55 minutes

Serves 4

4 large portobello
  mushrooms, stems
  removed

1 large red onion, thinly
  sliced

1 bunch fresh basil

1 large tomato, thinly
  sliced

1 tablespoon ground
  oregano

Dash salt and pepper

1 tablespoon grapeseed
  oil

1 small onion, diced

2 cloves garlic, crushed

4 ounces mushrooms,
  sliced

1 cup quinoa

2 cups vegetable stock

½ teaspoon salt

Preheat oven to 400°F.

Place portobello mushrooms (gill-side up) on a baking sheet.

Layer red onion slices, basil leaves, and tomato slices onto the mushrooms.

Sprinkle each portobello mushroom with dried oregano, salt, and pepper.

Place in oven and bake for 30–40 minutes until mushrooms are tender.

Heat the grapeseed oil in a large pan on medium-low heat.

Add the small onion and cook for about 5 minutes until transparent.

Stir in quinoa, vegetable stock, and salt and bring to a boil. Once boiling, reduce heat, cover, and simmer for 15 minutes.

Serve quinoa together with a portobello mushroom.

VEGETARIAN MAIN COURSES

Chana Masala

Total prep and cooking time: 45 minutes

Serves 6

1 cup brown rice

1 tablespoon coconut oil

2 medium onions, peeled and minced

2 cloves garlic, peeled and minced

1 tablespoon ground coriander

2 teaspoons ground cumin

½ teaspoon ground cayenne pepper

1 teaspoon ground turmeric

1 medium tomato, chopped

4 cups cooked chickpeas or 2 (15 oz.) cans chickpeas, rinsed and drained

1 cup vegetable broth

2 teaspoons paprika

1 teaspoon garam masala

½ teaspoon salt

½ lemon, juiced

2 teaspoons grated fresh ginger

4 cups fresh spinach

Add rice to a boiling pot of water. Cover and simmer for 45 minutes or until desired tenderness is reached.

Heat coconut oil in a large skillet. Add onions and garlic and sauté over medium heat until browned (3–5 minutes).

Turn heat to medium-low.

Add the coriander, cumin, cayenne, and turmeric. Stir for a few seconds.

Add the tomatoes and stir.

Cook the tomatoes until lightly browned.

Add chickpeas and a cup of vegetable broth and stir.

Add the paprika, garam masala, salt, and lemon juice.

Cook covered for 10 minutes.

Remove the cover and add the ginger. Stir and cook uncovered for another 30 seconds.

Serve warm over a bed of fresh spinach and brown rice.

Tip: Instead of using individual spices, you can use a chana masala spice mix, found in most Indian grocery stores.

VEGETARIAN MAIN COURSES

Green Lentil Salad

Total prep and cooking time: 45 minutes

Serves 4

2 cups dried green lentils

3 cups vegetable stock

2 onions, chopped

2 red peppers, thinly sliced

1 bunch cilantro, chopped

1 spring onion, chopped

1 carrot, shredded

3 prawns (optional)

4 cups leafy salad greens

Salad Dressing

3 tablespoons lemon juice

¼ cup olive oil

3 tablespoons balsamic vinegar

Salt and pepper, to taste

Rinse lentils and place in a large pot.

Add vegetable stock and onions to the lentils and bring to a boil. Once it boils, reduce heat and simmer for about 15 minutes or until lentils are tender.

Meanwhile, combine lemon juice, olive oil, and balsamic vinegar in a small bowl and mix thoroughly. Set aside.

Combine red peppers, cilantro, spring onion, and carrot in a large bowl.

If you want to add prawns, place in a small pan and cook with garlic for a couple of minutes, until they turn white.

Once lentils are tender, remove from heat and drain off remaining broth. Let cool.

Place lentils in a large bowl and top with carrot, red pepper, cilantro, spring onion, leafy salad greens, and prawns (optional).

Pour dressing over salad and serve immediately.

VEGETARIAN MAIN COURSES

Grilled Vegetables with Brown Rice

Total prep and cooking time: 55 minutes

Serves 4

1½ cups brown rice

3 peppers (yellow, red, and green), deseeded and cut into quarters

2 medium red onions, sliced

3 portobello mushrooms, sliced

2 small zucchinis, cut in half lengthways and sliced thinly

Olive oil, for brushing

2 tablespoons fresh thyme, chopped

Dressing

2 tablespoons olive oil

2 tablespoons lemon juice

2 cloves garlic, crushed

Salt and pepper, to taste

Place brown rice in a pot with water. Bring to a boil, and then simmer for 45 minutes or until tender.

Mix together the dressing. Set aside.

Arrange vegetables on a grill rack. Brush with olive oil and grill for 8–10 minutes or until tender and slightly brown.

Drain the rice and place in a bowl. Pour half the dressing over the top.

Add the vegetables on top, and then pour over the remaining dressing.

Garnish with chopped thyme.

VEGETARIAN MAIN COURSES

Vegetarian Chili

Total prep and cooking time: 45 minutes

Serves 6–8

1 tablespoon grapeseed oil

1 chopped onion

3 cloves minced garlic

2 tomatoes, diced, or 1 can organic diced tomatoes

2 carrots, cut into quarter-moons

2 stalks celery, sliced

10 mushrooms, sliced

2 tablespoons chili powder

2 teaspoons ground cumin

¼ teaspoon ground cloves

2 teaspoons unsweetened cocoa powder

3 cups black beans or kidney beans (cooked or canned)

1 cup water

2 tablespoons organic tomato paste

1 teaspoon sea salt

4 cups fresh spinach

Heat grapeseed oil in a large, heavy pan.

Add onions and garlic and sauté for 5 minutes.

Add the rest of the vegetables, chili powder, and cumin.

Sauté for another 5 minutes.

Add the rest of the ingredients (except spinach) and cook on low to medium heat for 30 minutes.

Serve warm on a bed of spinach.

Lemon and Dill Halibut

Total prep and cooking time: 20 minutes

Serves 4

4 halibut fish fillets
Dash sea salt
Dash black pepper
½ cup fresh dill, finely chopped
1 tablespoon fresh lemon juice

Rinse fish under cold water.

Season with salt and pepper.

Fill a skillet with ½–1 inch of water and heat until steaming.

Place fish in the skillet and top with dill.

Cook until fish is soft and flaking (about 5–7 minutes).

Squeeze lemon juice over fish, remove from heat, and serve immediately.

Serve with your choice of Happy Hormones side dishes.

MEAT, POULTRY, AND FISH MAIN COURSES

Tilapia with Roasted Red Pepper and Mango Salsa

Total prep and cooking time: 1 hour 15 minutes

Serves 4

Brown Rice

1 cup brown rice

2 cups water or vegetable stock

Salad

5 cups mixed salad greens

1 tomato, cut into ½-inch pieces

1 avocado, cut into ½-inch pieces

½ cucumber, cut into half-moons

3 green onions, sliced thinly

¼–½ teaspoon white sugar

Pinch salt

Drizzle white vinegar

Mango Salsa

2 red peppers, roasted

2 mangoes, diced

1 small red onion, diced

½ jalapeño (if desired), minced

¾ cup cilantro, chopped

Juice of ½ lime

Salt and pepper (to taste)

Fish

1 tablespoon grapeseed oil

4 tilapia fillets

MEAT, POULTRY, AND FISH MAIN COURSES

Place rice with 2 cups of water or vegetable broth into a pot and bring to a boil. Cover, reduce heat, and simmer for 45 minutes until rice is cooked to desired tenderness.

Turn on the broiler inside your oven and move rack to highest position. Put the red peppers directly onto the rack and allow skin to blacken. Turn peppers until most of the skin is charred.

Place peppers into a bowl and cover with plastic wrap. After 10–15 minutes, the skin can be peeled off under running water. Remove seeds and ribs and chop into small pieces for your salsa.

Toss mango, roasted peppers, red onion, jalapeño (optional), and cilantro with the lime juice and season with salt and pepper.

Place all of your salad ingredients into a bowl and mix well.

Sprinkle sugar and salt over the salad and drizzle with vinegar. Toss together.

Heat your grill. If you are using a barbecue, drizzle grapeseed oil onto a bed of aluminum foil and place fish fillets on top. If you are using a grill pan, lightly oil it with grapeseed oil. Grill fish until opaque (cooking time varies, depending on thickness of fish).

Serve fish hot on a bed of rice, garnished with salsa and the side salad.

MEAT, POULTRY, AND FISH MAIN COURSES

MEAT, POULTRY, AND FISH MAIN COURSES

Chicken Fajitas

Total prep and cooking time: 30 minutes

Serves 4

Fajita Mixture

1½ pounds chicken breast, cut into strips, ¼-inch thick

2 tablespoons grape seed oil

2 medium red onions, sliced lengthwise

3 bell peppers of various colors, sliced into ¼-inch strips

2 cups fresh spinach

8–12 soft corn tortillas

2 avocados, chopped

2 tomatoes, chopped

2 cups mixed salad greens

1 jalapeño (if you like spice), minced (optional)

Fajita Marinade

Juice of 1 lime

3 tablespoons olive oil

1 clove garlic, minced

½ teaspoon salt

½ teaspoon ground cumin

½ teaspoon chili powder

½ jalapeño, seeded and minced

¼ cup chopped cilantro

Combine marinade ingredients in a large bowl. Add chicken strips and coat well. Allow to marinate for 45 minutes.

Heat grapeseed oil in a large pan over high heat and cook your chicken strips until they are three-fourths of the way done (about 4–5 minutes).

Add the onion and pepper strips and cook until onions are soft and fragrant.

Add in spinach and heat until wilted.

Serve in corn tortillas with avocado, tomato, salad greens, and jalapeño (if using).

Serve with your choice of Happy Hormones side dishes.

MEAT, POULTRY, AND FISH MAIN COURSES

Roasted Chicken with Balsamic Vinaigrette

Total prep and cooking time: 2½ hours

Serves 8

1 whole organic chicken

Salt and freshly ground black pepper

1 large sweet onion, chopped

5 fresh figs, quartered

¼ cup balsamic vinegar

¼ cup extra virgin olive oil

1 tablespoon Dijon mustard

2 cloves garlic, crushed

1 tablespoon maple syrup

Fresh rosemary sprigs

Preheat oven to 475°F.

Rinse chicken under cold running water. Place chicken into a large baking dish or roasting pan. Sprinkle with salt and freshly ground black pepper.

Place half of the chopped onion inside the chicken cavity and the other half scattered along the bottom of the pan.

Place the figs around the chicken.

Whisk together the balsamic vinegar, olive oil, Dijon mustard, garlic, and maple syrup in a small bowl or cup. Pour over the chicken.

Place a few fresh rosemary sprigs on and around the chicken.

Add about ¼ cup of water to the bottom of the pan.

Place in the oven and roast at 475°F for about 20 minutes to seal in the juices. Reduce heat to 325°F and continue to cook until juices run clear (about another 1½ hours).

Serve with your choice of Happy Hormones side dishes.

MEAT, POULTRY, AND FISH MAIN COURSES

Grilled Steak with Vegetable Skewers

Total prep and cooking time: 30 minutes

Serves 3–4

1 pound sirloin steak

1 cup quinoa

2 cups water

2 colored peppers, sliced into quarters

2 small zucchinis, chopped into ½-inch rounds

1 large onion, chopped into ½-inch rounds

12 mushrooms, whole

1 tablespoon grapeseed oil

Salt and pepper (to taste)

Marinade

⅓ cup cooking sherry

⅓ cup tamari soy sauce

⅓ cup oil

2 tablespoons honey

2 tablespoons grated ginger root

2 cloves garlic, minced

Combine marinade ingredients in a small jar and shake to combine.

Cut steak into 2-inch cubes and place in a container. Pour over marinade and let marinate for 2–24 hours.

Pour off excess marinade and skewer steak pieces before grilling.

Place quinoa and water into a pot and bring to a boil. Cover, reduce heat to a simmer, and cook for 15 minutes until quinoa is tender.

Combine vegetables in a bowl, lightly drizzle with oil, and season with salt and pepper.

Heat grill or barbecue, and grill steak skewers to desired wellness. Remove from heat and cover with aluminum foil while vegetables get their turn.

Place vegetables on the grill, and grill until desired tenderness.

MEAT, POULTRY, AND FISH MAIN COURSES

Thai Green Curry

Total prep and cooking time: 45 minutes

Serves 4

1 cup brown rice

2 tablespoons green curry paste (recipe follows)

1 tablespoon grapeseed oil

1 (15 oz.) can coconut milk

1 pound flank steak, cut into 1-inch pieces

1 teaspoon lime juice

1 red bell pepper, diced

1 medium zucchini, cut in half lengthwise, and then into half-moons

1 tablespoon brown sugar

1 teaspoon fish sauce

¼ cup Thai basil leaves

4 cups spinach

Green Curry Paste

4 small green Thai chilies, or 1–2 jalapeño peppers

¼ cup red onion, diced

4 cloves garlic, minced

1 thumb-size piece fresh ginger, grated

1 stalk fresh lemongrass, minced

½ teaspoon ground coriander

½ teaspoon ground cumin

1 cup fresh cilantro leaves and stems, chopped

3 tablespoons fish sauce

1 teaspoon brown sugar

2 tablespoons lime juice

In a food processor or blender, combine the curry paste ingredients until a paste forms. If necessary, add a splash of water or coconut milk.

Place rice in a pot with 2 cups of water and bring to a boil. Once boiling, cover and reduce heat.

Simmer for 45 minutes until rice reaches the desired tenderness.

Combine 2 tablespoons of green curry paste with the grapeseed oil over medium heat and cook until fragrant. Add ½ cup of coconut milk and stir until the oil comes to the surface.

Add the steak and lime juice and continue cooking until the steak is almost done.

Add the red pepper, zucchini, remaining coconut milk, brown sugar, and fish sauce. Bring to a boil.

Add the basil, stir, and remove from heat.

Serve over a bed of spinach and brown rice.

MEAT, POULTRY, AND FISH MAIN COURSES

Honey Gingered Salmon

Total prep and cooking time: 75 minutes

Serves 4

4 salmon fillets

1 teaspoon ground ginger

1 teaspoon garlic powder

⅓ cup tamari

3 tablespoons freshly squeezed orange juice

3 tablespoons honey

1 green onion, chopped

Place salmon in a large dish.

Combine ginger, garlic, tamari, orange juice, honey, and green onion and mix well.

Pour over the salmon.

Cover the salmon and refrigerate for 1 hour.

Preheat a grill to medium heat and lightly oil to prevent the fish from sticking to the grill.

Remove the salmon from the fridge, discarding any excess marinade.

Grill salmon for 12–15 minutes per inch of thickness or until the fish flakes easily with a fork.

Serve with your choice of Happy Hormones side dishes.

Tabbouleh

Total prep and cooking time: 40 minutes

Serves 6

1 cup quinoa

2 cups water

1 (15 oz.) can garbanzo beans

½ cup parsley, chopped

1 bunch mint, chopped

2 medium cucumbers, chopped

2 tomatoes, chopped

3 tablespoons lemon juice

4 tablespoons extra virgin olive oil

Sea salt (to taste)

Place quinoa in a pot and add 2 cups of water. Bring to a boil.

Reduce heat to low and simmer covered for 20 minutes or until quinoa reaches the desired tenderness.

Fluff with a fork, cover, and let sit for another 10 minutes.

Rinse the garbanzo beans and set aside.

Place garbanzo beans, parsley, mint, cucumber, and tomato in a large bowl. Add quinoa once cooled and combine with other ingredients.

Mix the lemon juice and olive oil in a small bowl and pour over the quinoa and vegetable mixture. Gently mix and salt to taste.

Ginger and Garlic Collard Greens

Total prep and cooking time: 20 minutes

Serves 4

SIDES

2 bunches mixed collard greens, chopped

2 cloves garlic, finely chopped

2 teaspoons ginger, finely chopped

2 teaspoons tamari

2 teaspoons olive oil

Fill a large pot with ½ inch of water and heat to high.

Add mixed collard greens and cook for 3 minutes until desired tenderness is reached.

In a frying pan sauté garlic and ginger for 30 seconds until golden brown.

Strain greens through a colander and transfer to a bowl.

Add the sautéed garlic, ginger, tamari, and olive oil and mix well.

Collard Greens with
Toasted Pine Nuts and Raisins

Total prep and cooking time: 20 minutes

Serves 6

⅓ cup pine nuts

1 tablespoon grapeseed oil

2 bunches mixed collard greens, chopped

½ teaspoon sea salt

¼ cup raisins

Preheat oven to 350°F.

Place pine nuts on a baking tray and toast for 5 minutes or until light brown. Set aside and let cool.

Heat grapeseed oil in a pan.

Add collard greens, sea salt, and raisins. Stir and cook for 5 minutes.

Turn off heat, add in pine nuts, and transfer to serving dish.

SIDES

Warm Broccoli and Avocado Salad

Total prep and cooking time: 20 minutes

Serves 6

2 bunches broccoli, chopped

2 tablespoons fresh lemon juice

1 tablespoon olive oil

¼ teaspoon sea salt

1 avocado, chopped

Fill a pot with 1 inch of water and steam broccoli for 7–10 minutes or until tender.

In a mixing bowl, combine the lemon juice, olive oil, and salt. Add the avocado and warm broccoli. Mix and serve.

Sautéed Brussels Sprouts with Cranberries

Total prep and cooking time: 15 minutes

Serves 6

2 tablespoons grapeseed oil

1 small red onion, thinly sliced

⅓ cup slivered almonds

2 pounds Brussels sprouts, halved

½ teaspoon sea salt

⅓ cup dried cranberries

½ cup water

Freshly ground black pepper

Heat grapeseed oil in a large pot.

Add red onion and sauté for 2 minutes.

Add slivered almonds, Brussels sprouts, and sea salt. Sauté for another 5 minutes.

Add the dried cranberries and water.

Cook covered, stirring occasionally for 5–10 minutes until desired tenderness is reached.

Season with freshly ground black pepper and serve.

Almond and Raisin Coleslaw

Total prep and cooking time: 15 minutes

Serves 6

3 cups green cabbage, sliced

2 cups red cabbage, sliced

4 carrots, grated

¾ cup fresh chives, chopped

¾ cup chopped almonds

½ cup raisins

Dressing

6 tablespoons olive oil

4 tablespoons apple cider vinegar

1 tablespoon honey

1 teaspoon Dijon mustard

½ teaspoon sea salt

Combine cabbage, carrots, chives, almonds, and raisins in a large mixing bowl. Mix well.

Whisk ingredients for the dressing in a small bowl. Pour over the vegetables and mix well.

Cucumber Tomato and Basil Salad

Total prep and cooking time: 15 minutes

Serves 4

1 large cucumber, sliced

3 tomatoes, quartered, and then sliced

½ cup fresh basil, thinly sliced

2 cloves fresh garlic, finely chopped

2 tablespoons olive oil

2 tablespoons red wine vinegar

Sea salt and freshly ground black pepper (to taste)

Place all ingredients into a large bowl and mix together. Add salt and pepper to taste. Gently toss and serve immediately.

SIDES

Fruit and Nut Bars

Total cooking and prep time: 30 minutes

3½ cups almonds

1 teaspoon sea salt

2 teaspoons vanilla extract

4 cups dried unsweetened pineapple, chopped

4 cups pitted dates

1½ cups shredded coconut

Combine almonds, salt, and vanilla in a food processor. Process into a fine powder.

Slowly add chopped pineapple and dates. Mix well.

Transfer to a large bowl and add in the coconut. Mix well.

Form into 2-inch bars.

Refrigerate and serve.

Store any extras in the freezer.

Kale Chips

Total cooking and prep time: 20 minutes

Serves 20 or more

2 bunches kale

2 tablespoons olive oil

1 teaspoon cayenne pepper

½ teaspoon salt

1 teaspoon paprika powder

Preheat oven to 350°F.

Remove kale leaves from stalk, leaving them in large pieces.

Toss the leaves with olive oil.

Place the kale leaves on a baking pan in a single layer.

Bake for 10–12 minutes or until leaves start to brown.

Remove from oven and sprinkle with cayenne, salt, and paprika powder.

Mixed Berries with Pumpkin Seeds

Total prep time: 10 minutes

Serves 1

1 tablespoon pumpkin seeds
¾ cup fresh berries

Sprinkle pumpkin seeds over berries. Enjoy.

Toasted Nut Mix

Total cooking and prep time: 20 minutes

Serves 8

½ cup walnuts, raw and unsalted

½ cup almonds, raw and unsalted

½ cup pecans, raw and unsalted

½ cup cashews, raw and unsalted

2 teaspoons coconut oil

2 teaspoons maple syrup

1 tablespoon garam masala

1 teaspoon sea salt

Preheat oven to 300°F.

In a bowl mix together nuts, oil, and maple syrup.

Place mixture on a baking sheet and roast in the oven until lightly browned (about 10–15 minutes).

Remove from heat and toss with garam masala and salt.

SNACKS

Guacamole with Rice Crackers

Total prep time: 20 minutes

Serves 4

2 avocados, cut in half, with seeds removed

½ small red onion, finely chopped

1 small tomato, finely chopped

¼ cup cilantro, chopped

Juice of 1 lime

½ teaspoon sea salt and pepper

Rice crackers

Combine all ingredients in a mixing bowl and mash the avocado with a fork until smooth.

Dip crackers and enjoy.

Celery Sticks with Almond Butter

Total prep time: 10 minutes

Serves 1

2 stalks celery

1 tablespoon almond butter

Wash and cut celery into 3-inch sticks.

Fill celery with almond butter.

References

What Are Hormones and Why Are They Important?

Altern Med Rev. 2000; 5(4):306-33.

Barnes, BO, Galton. *Hypothyroidism: the unsuspected illness.* NY: Thomas Crowell, 1976.

Beers, MH, Porter, RS, Jones, TV. The Merck Manual of Diagnosis and Therapy. 18th ed. 2006. Merck Publishing Group.

Blanchard. K. *The Functional Approach to Hypothyroidism.* NY. Hatherleigh Press. 2012.

Cooper DS. Subclinical hypothyroidism. Advances in Endocrinology and Metabolism. 1991; 2; 77.

Gardner DG, Shoback D. *Greenspan's Basic & Clinical Endocrinology,* 8th ed. New York: McGraw-Hill Medical, 2007.

Hertoghe, T. *The Hormone Solution*. NY. Three Rivers Press. 2002.

Hudson, Tori. *Women's Encyclopedia of Natural Medicine*. NY. McGraw Hill. 2008.

Kelly, GS. Peripheral metabolism of thyroid hormones: a review.

Kharrazian, D. *Why do I still have thyroid symptoms when my lab tests are normal*. CA: Elephant Printing, 2010.

Tilgner, S. *Herbal Medicine From the Heart of the Earth*. OR. Wise Acres Press. 1999.

Tsigos, C, Chrouos, GP. Hypothalamic–pituitary–adrenal axis, neuroendocrine factors and stress. *Journal of Psychosomatic Research*. 2002; 53(4): 865-871

Weetman AP. Hypothyroidism: screening and subclinical disease. *British Medical Journal*. 1997; 19: 1175-1178.

Wilson, J. *Adrenal Fatigue the 21st Century Stress Syndrome*. CA. Smart Publications. 2001.

Symptoms of Hormonal Imbalances

Aardel-Eriksson, E, Thorell, LH. Salivary cortisol, posttraumatic stress symptoms and general health in the acute phase and during 9 month follow-up. *Biol Psychiatry*. 2001; 50(12): 986-993.

Arlt, W, et al. Dehydroepiandrosterone replacement in women with adrenal insufficiency pharmacokinetics, bio-conversion and clinical effects on well-being, sexuality and cognition. *Endocr Res.* 2000; 26(4): 505-511.

Asthana, S, et al. High dose estradiol improves cognition for women with AD: results of a randomized study, *Neurology.* 2001; 57(4): 605-612.

Barnes, BO, Galton. *Hypothyroidism: the unsuspected illness.* NY: Thomas Crowell, 1976.

Beers, MH, Porter, RS, Jones, TV. The Merck Manual of Diagnosis and Therapy. 18th ed. 2006. Merck Publishing Group.

Bernini, GP, et al. Influence of endogenous androgens on carotid wall in postmenopausal women. *Menopause:* 2001; 8(1): 43-50.

Blanchard. K. *The Functional Approach to Hypothyroidism.* NY. Hatherleigh Press. 2012.

Buchanan, JR, et al. Effect of excess endogenous androgens on bone density in young women. *J Clin Endocrinol Metab.* 1998; 67(5): 937.

Chrouos, GP. The role of stress and the hypothalamic-pituitary-adrenal axis in the pathogenesis of the metabolic syndrome: neuroendocrine and target tissue-related causes. *Int J Obes Relat Metab Discord.* 2000; Jun; 24(2): S50-S55.

Cleare, AJ, et al. Hypothalamo-pituitary-adrenal axis dysfunction in chronic fatigue syndrome, and the effects of low dose hydrocortisone therapy. *J Clin Endocrinol Metab*. 2001; 86(8): 3545-3554.

Cleghorn, RA. Adrenal cortisol insufficiency: psychological and neurological observations. *Canad Med Ass J*. 1951; 65: 449.

Cooper DS. Subclinical hypothyroidism. Advances in Endocrinology and Metabolism. 1991; 2; 77.

Davis, S.R. The clinical use of androgens in female sexual disorders. *J Sex Marital Ther*. 1998; 24(3): 153-156.

De Lignieres, B, et al. Differential effects of exogenous estradiol and progesterone on mood in postmenopausal women: individual dose/effect relationship. *Maturitas*. 1982; 4: 67-72.

Demitrack MA. *Evidence for impaired activation of the hypothalamic-pituitary-adrenal axis in patients with chronic fatigue syndrome*. J. Clin Endocrinol Metab. 1991;73:1244-1234.

Deutsch, S, et al. The correlation of serum estrogens and androgens with bone density in late postmenopause. *Int J Gynaecol Obstet*. 1987; 25(3): 217-222.

Fingerova, H, et al. Reduced serum dehydroepiandrosterone levels in postmenopausal osteoporosis. *Ceska Gynekol*. 1998; 63(2): 110-113.

Freeman, EW, et al. Anxiolytic metabolites of progesterone: correlation with mood and performance measures following oral progesterone administration to healthy female volunteers. *Neuroendocrinology*. 1993; 58(4): 478-484.

Gardner DG, Shoback D. *Greenspan's Basic & Clinical Endocrinology*, 8th ed. New York: McGraw-Hill Medical, 2007.

Gold, PW, Chrousos, GP. Organization of the stress system and its dysregulation in melancholic and atypical depression: high vs. low CRH/NE states. *Mol Psychiatry*. 2002; 7(3): 254-175.

Greenspan SG, Gardner DG. Basic and Clinical Endocrinology. 6th ed. CT. Appleton and Lange. 2001.

Guay, A.T, Decreased testosterone in regularly menstruation women with decreased libido: a clinical observation. *J Sex Marital Ther*. 2001; 27(5): 513-519.

Hertoghe, T. *The Hormone Solution*. NY. Three Rivers Press. 2002.

Holick, MF. Sunlight and vitamin D for bone health and prevention of autoimmune diseases, cancers, and cardiovascular disease. *Am J Clin Nutr*. December 2004; 80(6)

Kenny, AM, et al. Effects of transdermal testosterone on bone and muscle in older men with low bioavailable testosterone levels. *J Gerontol A Biol Sci Med Sci*. 2001;56(5)266-272.

Kharrazian, D. *Why do I still have thyroid symptoms when my lab tests are normal.* CA: Elephant Printing, 2010.

Labrie, F, et al. Effect of 12 month dehydroepiandrosterone replacement therapy on bone, vagina and endometrium in postmenopausal women. *J Clin Endocrinol Metab.* 1997; 82(10): 3498-3505.

Negata, C, et al. Association of dehydroepiandrosterone sulfate with serum HDL cholesterol concentrations in post-menopausal Japanese women. *Maturitas.* 1998; 31(1): 21-27.

Peters, EM, Anderson, R, Nieman, DC, et al. Vitamin C supplementation attenuates the increases in circulating cortisol, adrenaline and anti-inflammatory polypeptides following ultramarathon running. *Int J Sports Med.* 2001; 22(7): 537-543.

Rothenberg, R, Hart, K. Hormone Optimization in Preventative/Regenerative Medicine. Panda Press. CA.

Selye, H. *The stress of life.* NY: McGraw-Hill. 1956

Smith, YR, et al. Long term estrogen replacement is associated with improved nonverbal memory and attentional measures in postmenopausal women. *Fertil Steril.* 2001; 76(6): 1101-1107.

Smith, YR, et al. Long term estrogen replacement is associated with improved nonverbal memory and attentional measures in postmenopausal women. *Feril Steril*. 2001; 76(6): 1101-1107.

Stowe, RP, Pierson, Dl, Barrett, AD. Elevated stress hormone levels relate to Epstein-Barr virus reactivation in astronauts. *Psychosom Med*. 2001; 63(6): 891-895.

Straub, RH, Herfarth, H, Falk, W, et al. Uncoupling of the sympathetic nervous system and the hypothalamic-pituitary-adrenal axis in inflammatory bowel disease? *Neuroimmunol*. 2002; 126(1-2): 116-125.

Tintera, JW. *Hypoadrenocorticism*. NY: Adrenal Metabolic Research Society. 1956

Tsigos, C, Chrouos, GP. Hypothalamic–pituitary–adrenal axis, neuroendocrine factors and stress. *Journal of Psychosomatic Research*. 2002; 53(4): 865-871

Tsigos, C, Chrousos, GP. Physiology of the hypothalamic-pituitary-adrenal axis in health and dysregulation in psychiatric and autoimmune disorders. *Endocrinol Metab Clin North Am*. 1994; Sept; 23(3): 451-466.

Van den Berghe, G. The neuroendocrine response to stress is a dynamic process. *Best Pract Res Clin Endocrinol Metab*. 2001; Dec; 15.

Wang, C, et al. Transdermal testosterone gel improves sexual function, mood, muscle strength, and body composition parameters in hypogonadal men. *J Clin Endocrinol Metab.* 2000; 85(8): 2839-2853.

Weetman AP. Hypothyroidism: screening and subclinical disease. *British Medical Journal.* 1997;19: 1175-1178.

Wilson, J. *Adrenal Fatigue the 21st Century Stress Syndrome.* CA. Smart Publications. 2001.

Nutrition for Happy Hormones

Anderson, JW. Dietary Fibre, complex carbohydrate and coronary artery disease. *Can J Cardiol.* 1995; 11: 55G-62G.

Fruedenheim, JL, et al. Premenopausal breast cancer risk and intake of vegetables, fruit and related nutrients. *J Natl Cancer Inst.* 1996; 88: 340-348.

Fuyns, A. Alcohol and Cancer. *Proc Nutr Soc.* 1990; 49: 145-151.

Ginsburg, E. Effects of alcohol ingestion on estrogen in postmenopausal women. *JAMA.* 1996; 276(21): 1747-1751.

Holick, MF. Sunlight and vitamin D for bone health and prevention of autoimmune diseases, cancers, and cardiovascular disease. *Am J Clin Nutr.* December 2004; 80(6)

Ingram, DM, et al. Effect of low fat diet on female sex hormone levels. *J Natl Cancer Inst.* 1987; 79(6): 1225-1229.

Marz, R. Medical Nutrition From Marz. 2nd ed. Omni-press. OR. 1999.

Pitchford, P. Healing with Whole Foods. Revised Edition. North Atlantic Books. CA. 1993.

Natural Solutions for Estrogen Excess and Deficiency

Anderson, JW. Dietary Fibre, complex carbohydrate and coronary artery disease. *Can J Cardiol.* 1995; 11: 55G-62G.

Bone, K. *The Ultimate Herbal Compendium.* Australia. Phytotherapy Press. 2007.

Dalton, K. The premenstrual syndrome and progesterone therapy. Chicago IL: Year Book Pub. 1977.

Deutsch, S, et al. The correlation of serum estrogens and androgens with bone density in late postmenopause. *Int J Gynaecol Obstet.* 1987; 25(3): 217-222.

Duker, E, et al. Effects of Extracts from *Cimicifuga racemosa* on gonadotropin release in menopausal women and ovariectomized rats. Plant Med. 1991; 57; 420-424.

Greenspan SG, Gardner DG. Basic and Clinical Endocrinology. 6th ed. CT. Appleton and Lange. 2001.

Hansel, R. Phytopharmaka. 2nd ed. Berlin: Springer Verlag; 1991;223-230.

Herous O, Peter D, Heggtevelt HA. Long term effect of suboptimal magnesium and calcium contents of organs on cold intolerance and life span , and the pathological consequences in rats. *Journal of Nutrition*. 1997;107:1640

Holick, MF. Sunlight and vitamin D for bone health and prevention of autoimmune diseases, cancers, and cardiovascular disease. *Am J Clin Nutr*. December 2004; 80(6)

Horrobin DF. The role of essential fatty acids and prostaglandins in premenstrual syndrome. *Journal of Reproductive Medicine*. 1983; 28:465

Hudson, Tori. *Women's Encyclopedia of Natural Medicine*. NY. McGraw Hill. 2008.

Kotsopoulos, J, et al. Relationship between caffeine intake and plasma sex hormone concentrations in premenopausal and postmenopausal women. *Cancer*. 2009; 115(12): 2765-74.

Lee, JR. What your doctor may not tell you about menopause. NY: Warner Books. 1996.

Marz, R. Medical Nutrition From Marz. 2nd ed. Omni-press. OR. 1999.

Mayo, JL. A Natural Approach to Menopause. *Clin Nutr Insights*. 1997; 7: 1-8.

Rothenberg, R, Hart, K. Hormone Optimization in Preventative/Regenerative Medicine. Panda Press. CA.

Sherwood, RA, et al. Magnesium and the premenstrual syndrome. *Ann Clin Biochem.* 1986; 23: 667.

Smith, YR, et al. Long term estrogen replacement is associated with improved nonverbal memory and attentional measures in postmenopausal women. *Fertil Steril.* 2001; 76(6): 1101-1107.

Tabakova P, Dimitrov M, Ognyanov K, Popvassilev N. "Clinical study of Tribestan in females with endocrine sterility." Unpublished. tribestan.com.

Tilgner, S. *Herbal Medicine From the Heart of the Earth.* OR. Wise Acres Press. 1999.

Wimalawansa, SJ, et al. The effect of percutaneous estradiol and low dose human calcitonin on postmenopausal vertebral bone loss. *Osteoporosis.* 1987; 528-532.

Natural Solutions for Progesterone Deficiency

Bone, K. *The Ultimate Herbal Compendium.* Australia. Phytotherapy Press. 2007.

Dalton, K. The premenstrual syndrome and progesterone therapy. Chicago IL: Year Book Pub. 1977.

Freeman, EW, et al. Anxiolytic metabolites of progesterone: correlation with mood and performance measures following oral progesterone administration to healthy female volunteers. *Neuroendocrinology*. 1993; 58(4): 478-484.

Herous O, Peter D, Heggtevelt HA. Long term effect of suboptimal magnesium and calcium contents of organs on cold intolerance and life span , and the pathological consequences in rats. *Journal of Nutrition*. 1997;107:1640

Holick, MF. Sunlight and vitamin D for bone health and prevention of autoimmune diseases, cancers, and cardiovascular disease. *Am J Clin Nutr*. December 2004; 80(6)

Horrobin, DF. The role of essential fatty acids and prostaglandins in premenstrual syndrome. *Journal of Reproductive Medicine*. 1983; 28:465

Hudson, Tori. *Women's Encyclopedia of Natural Medicine*. NY. McGraw Hill. 2008.

Lee, JR. What your doctor may not tell you about menopause. NY: Warner Books. 1996.

Marz, R. Medical Nutrition From Marz. 2nd ed. Omni-press. OR. 1999.

Peters, JR, Walker, RF, Riad-Fahmy, D, Hall, R. *Salivary cortisol assays for assessing pituitary-adrenal reserve*. Clin Endocrinol. 1982. 17;6: 583-592.

Rothenberg, R, Hart K. Hormone Optimization in Preventative/Regenerative Medicine. Panda Press. CA.

Saden-Krehula, M, et al. Delta-3-ketosteroids in the Flowers and Leaves of *Vitex agnus-castus*. *Planta Med*. 1990; 56: 547.

Sherwood, RA, et al. Magnesium and the premenstrual syndrome. *Ann Clin Biochem*. 1986; 23: 667.

Sliutz, G, et al. *Agnus-castus* extracts inhibit prolactin secretion of rat pituitary cells. *Horm Metab Res*. 1993; 25(5): 253-255.

Tilgner, S. *Herbal Medicine From the Heart of the Earth*. OR. Wise Acres Press. 1999.

Wilson, J. *Adrenal Fatigue the 21st Century Stress Syndrome*. CA. Smart Publications. 2001.

Natural Solutions for Cortisol Excess and Deficiency

Bone, K. *The Ultimate Herbal Compendium*. Australia. Phytotherapy Press. 2007.

Brekham II, Kirillov OI. *Effect of* Eleutherococcus *on alarm phase of stress*. Life Science. 1969; 8(3): 113-121.

Bruneton, J. *Pharmacognosy, Phytochemistry, Medicinal Plants*. Paris: Lavoisier; 1995.

Cleare, AJ, et al. Hypothalamo-pituitary-adrenal axis dysfunction in chronic fatigue syndrome, and the effects of low dose hydrocortisone therapy. *J Clin Endocrinol Metab*. 2001; 86(8): 3545-3554.

Greenspan SG, Gardner DG. Basic and Clinical Endocrinology. 6th ed. CT. Appleton and Lange. 2001.

Holick, MF. Sunlight and vitamin D for bone health and prevention of autoimmune diseases, cancers, and cardiovascular disease. *Am J Clin Nutr*. December 2004; 80(6)

Hudson, Tori. *Women's Encyclopedia of Natural Medicine*. NY. McGraw Hill. 2008.

Jefferies, W. Safe Uses of Cortisone. IL. Thomas, 1981.

Kraemer, WJ, et al. Effects of heavy-resistance training on hormonal response patterns in younger vs. older men. *Journal of Applied Physiology*. 1999; 87(3): 982-992.

Marz, R. Medical Nutrition From Marz. 2nd ed. Omni-press. OR. 1999.

Peters, EM, Anderson, R, Nieman, DC, et al. Vitamin C supplementation attenuates the increases in circulating cortisol, adrenaline and anti-inflammatory polypeptides following ultramarathon running. *Int J Sports Med*. 2001; 22(7): 537-543.

Rothenberg, R, Hart K. Hormone Optimization in Preventative/Regenerative Medicine. Panda Press. CA.

Selye, H. *The stress of life*. NY: McGraw-Hill. 1956

Tilgner, S. *Herbal Medicine From the Heart of the Earth*. OR. Wise Acres Press. 1999.

Tsigos, C, Chrouos, GP. Hypothalamic–pituitary–adrenal axis, neuroendocrine factors and stress. *Journal of Psychosomatic Research*. 2002; 53(4): 865-871

Volek JS, Kraemer WJ, Bush JA, Incledon, T, Boetes, M. Testosterone and cortisol in relationship to dietary nutrients and resistance exercise. *Journal of Applied Physiology*. 1997; 82(1): 49-54.

Wilson, J. *Adrenal Fatigue the 21st Century Stress Syndrome*. CA. Smart Publications. 2001.

Natural Solutions for Low Thyroid

Barnes, BO, Galton. *Hypothyroidism: the unsuspected illness*. NY: Thomas Crowell, 1976.

Berry MJ, Larsen PR. The role of selenium in thyroid hormone action. *Endocrine Reviews*. 1992; 13: 207-220.

Blanchard. K. *The Functional Approach to Hypothyroidism*. NY. Hatherleigh Press. 2012.

Bone, K. *The Ultimate Herbal Compendium*. Australia. Phytotherapy Press. 2007.

Cooper DS. Subclinical hypothyroidism. Advances in Endocrinology and Metabolism. 1991; 2; 77.

Gardner DG, Shoback D. *Greenspan's Basic & Clinical Endocrinology*, 8th ed. New York: McGraw-Hill Medical, 2007.

Goodman, LS, Gilman A. The Pharmacological Basis of Therapeutics. 9th ed. MacMillan Pub. Co., NY, 1975.

Hertoghe, T. *The Hormone Solution.* NY. Three Rivers Press. 2002.

Holick, MF. Sunlight and vitamin D for bone health and prevention of autoimmune diseases, cancers, and cardiovascular disease. *Am J Clin Nutr.* December 2004; 80(6)

Hudson, Tori. *Women's Encyclopedia of Natural Medicine.* NY. McGraw Hill. 2008.

Kharrazian, D. *Why do I still have thyroid symptoms when my lab tests are normal.* CA: Elephant Printing, 2010.

Marz, R. Medical Nutrition From Marz. 2nd ed. Omni-press. OR. 1999.

Meinhold H, et al. Effects of iodine and selenium deficiency on iodothyronine deiodinases in brain, thyroid, and peripheral tissue. *JAMA.* 1992;19:8-12.

Nishiyama S, Futagoishi-Suginohara Y, Matsukura M, et al. Zinc supplementation alters thyroid hormone metabolism in disabled patients with zinc deficiency. *J Am Coll Nutr.* 1994;13;62-67.

Pizzorno JE, Murray MT. *Textbook of Natural Medicine*. Churchill Livingstone, NY, 1999.

Rothenberg, R, Hart, K. Hormone Optimization in Preventative/Regenerative Medicine. Panda Press. CA.

Tilgner, S. *Herbal Medicine From the Heart of the Earth*. OR. Wise Acres Press. 1999.

Weetman AP. Hypothyroidism: screening and subclinical disease. *British Medical Journal*. 1997;19: 1175-1178.

Wilson, J. *Adrenal Fatigue the 21st Century Stress Syndrome*. CA. Smart Publications. 2001.

Natural Solutions for DHEA Deficiency

Bone, K. *The Ultimate Herbal Compendium*. Australia. Phytotherapy Press. 2007.

Buchanan, JR, et al. Effect of excess endogenous androgens on bone density in young women. *J Clin Endocrinol Metab*. 1998; 67(5): 937.

Fingerova, H, et al. Reduced serum dehydroepiandrosterone levels in postmenopausal osteoporosis. *Ceska Gynekol*. 1998; 63(2): 110-113.

Holick, MF. Sunlight and vitamin D for bone health and prevention of autoimmune diseases, cancers, and cardiovascular disease. *Am J Clin Nutr.* December 2004; 80(6)

Hudson, Tori. *Women's Encyclopedia of Natural Medicine.* NY. McGraw Hill. 2008.

Labrie, F, et al. Effect of 12 month dehydroepiandrosterone replacement therapy on bone, vagina and endometrium in postmenopausal women. *J Clin Endocrinol Metab.* 1997; 82(10): 3498-3505.

Marz, R. Medical Nutrition From Marz. 2nd ed. Omni-press. OR. 1999.

Peters, EM, Anderson, R, Nieman, DC, et al. Vitamin C supplementation attenuates the increases in circulating cortisol, adrenaline and anti-inflammatory polypeptides following ultramarathon running. *Int J Sports Med.* 2001; 22(7): 537-543.

Rothenberg, R, Hart K. Hormone Optimization in Preventative/Regenerative Medicine. Panda Press. CA.

Tilgner, S. *Herbal Medicine From the Heart of the Earth.* OR. Wise Acres Press. 1999.

Tsigos, C, Chrouos, GP. Hypothalamic–pituitary–adrenal axis, neuroendocrine factors and stress. *Journal of Psychosomatic Research.* 2002; 53(4): 865-871

Tsigos, C, Chrouos, GP. Hypothalamic–pituitary–adrenal axis, neuroendocrine factors and stress. *Journal of Psychosomatic Research*. 2002; 53(4): 865-871

Wilson, J. *Adrenal Fatigue the 21st Century Stress Syndrome*. CA. Smart Publications. 2001.

Natural Solutions for Testosterone Deficiency

Bernini, GP, et al. Influence of endogenous androgens on carotid wall in postmenopausal women. *Menopause*: 2001; 8(1): 43-50.

Bone, K. *The Ultimate Herbal Compendium*. Australia. Phytotherapy Press. 2007.

Buchanan, JR, et al. Effect of excess endogenous androgens on bone density in young women. *J Clin Endocrinol Metab*. 1998; 67(5): 937.

Davis, S.R. The clinical use of androgens in female sexual disorders. *J Sex Marital Ther*. 1998; 24(3): 153-156.

El–Tantawy, WH, Temraz A, El–Gindi, OD. Free serum testosterone level in male rats treated with *Tribulus alatus* extracts. *Int Braz J Urol*. 2007; 33(4).

Fahim, MS, et al. Effect of *Panax* Ginseng on Testosterone Level and Prostate in Male Rats. *Systems Biology in Reproductive Medicine*. 1982; 8(4): 261-263

Guay, A.T, Decreased testosterone in regularly menstruation women with decreased libido: a clinical observation. *J Sex Marital Ther*. 2001; 27(5): 513-519.

Holick, MF. Sunlight and vitamin D for bone health and prevention of autoimmune diseases, cancers, and cardiovascular disease. *Am J Clin Nutr*. December 2004; 80(6)

Hudson, Tori. *Women's Encyclopedia of Natural Medicine*. NY. McGraw Hill. 2008.

Kenny, AM, et al. Effects of transdermal testosterone on bone and muscle in older men with low bioavailable testosterone levels. *J Gerontol A Biol Sci Med Sci*. 2001; 56(5): 266-272.

Kraemer, WJ, et al. Effects of heavy-resistance training on hormonal response patterns in younger vs. older men. *Journal of Applied Physiology*. 1999; 87(3): 982-992.

Marz, R. Medical Nutrition From Marz. 2nd ed. Omni-press. OR. 1999.

Rothenberg, R, Hart, K. Hormone Optimization in Preventative/Regenerative Medicine. Panda Press. CA.

Salvati G, Genovesi G, Marcellini L, Paolini P, De Nuccio I, Pepe M, Re M. Effects of *Panax* Ginseng C.A. Meyer saponins on male fertility. *Panminerva Med.* 1996; 38(4):249-54.

Sinclair, S. Male infertility: nutritional and environmental considerations. *Altern Med Rev.* 2000; 5(1): 28-38.

Snyder, PJ, et al. Effects of testosterone replacement in hypogonadal men. *J Clin Endocrinol Metab.* 2000: 85(8): 2670-2677.

Tilgner, S. *Herbal Medicine From the Heart of the Earth.* OR. Wise Acres Press. 1999.

Volek JS, Kraemer WJ, Bush JA, Incledon, T, Boetes, M. Testosterone and cortisol in relationship to dietary nutrients and resistance exercise. *Journal of Applied Physiology.* 1997; 82(1): 49-54.

Wang, C, et al. Transdermal testosterone gel improves sexual function, mood, muscle strength, and body composition parameters in hypogonadal men. *J Clin Endocrinol Metab.* 2000; 85(8): 2839-2853.

Wilson, J. *Adrenal Fatigue the 21st Century Stress Syndrome.* CA. Smart Publications. 2001.

Hormone Replacement Therapy

Arlt, W, et al. Dehydroepiandrosterone replacement in women with adrenal insufficiency pharmacokinetics, bioconversion and clinical effects on well-being, sexuality and cognition. *Endocr Res.* 2000; 26(4): 505-511.

Bernini, GP, et al. Influence of endogenous androgens on carotid wall in postmenopausal women. *Menopause:* 2001; 8(1): 43-50.

Buchanan, JR, et al. Effect of excess endogenous androgens on bone density in young women. *J Clin Endocrinol Metab.* 1998; 67(5): 937.

Canonico M, Plu-Bureau G, Lowe G, Scarabin PY. Hormone replacement therapy and risk of venous thromboembolism in postmenopausal women: systematic review and meta-analysis. *BMJ.* 2008;336:1227

Cleare, AJ, et al. Hypothalamo-pituitary-adrenal axis dysfunction in chronic fatigue syndrome, and the effects of low dose hydrocortisone therapy. *J Clin Endocrinol Metab.* 2001; 86(8): 3545-3554.

Cleghorn, R.A. Adrenal cortisol insufficiency: psychological and neurological observations. *Canad Med Ass J.* 1951; 65: 449.

Davis, S.R. The clinical use of androgens in female sexual disorders. *J Sex Marital Ther.* 1998; 24(3): 153-156.

De Lignieres, B, et al. Differential effects of exogenous estradiol and progesterone on mood in postmenopausal women: individual dose/effect relationship. *Maturitas.* 1982; 4: 67-72.

Deutsch, S, et al. The correlation of serum estrogens and androgens with bone density in late postmenopause. *Int J Gynaecol Obstet.* 1987; 25(3): 217-222.

Feldman, HA, et al. Low dehydroepiandrosterone sulfate and heart disease in middle-aged men: cross sectional results from Massachusetts Male Aging Study. *Ann Epidemiol:* 2001; 153(1): 79-89.

Fingerova, H, et al. Reduced serum dehydroepiandrosterone levels in postmenopausal osteoporosis. *Ceska Gynekol.* 1998; 63(2): 110-113.

Gerhard, M, et al. Estradiol therapy combined with progesterone and endothelium-dependent vasodilation in postmenopausal women. *Circulation:* 1998; 98(12): 1158-1163.

Guay, A.T, Decreased testosterone in regularly menstruation women with decreased libido: a clinical observation. *J Sex Marital Ther.* 2001; 27(5): 513-519.

Hanke, H, et al. Estradiol concentrations in premenopausal women with coronary heart disease. *Coron Artery Dis.* 1997; 8(8): 511-515.

Hargrove, JT, Osteen, KG. An Alternative Method of Hormone Replacement Therapy Using The Natural Sex Steroids. *Infer & Repr. Clinics N. Am.* 1995; 6(4): 654-660.

Holtorf, K. The Bioidentical Hormone Debate: Are Bioidentical Hormones (Estradiol, Estriol, and Progesterone) Safer or More Efficacious than Commonly Used Synthetic Versions in Hormone Replacement Therapy? *Postgraduate Medicine.* 2009;121(1).

Hudson, Tori. *Women's Encyclopedia of Natural Medicine.* NY. McGraw Hill. 2008.

Jefferies, W. Safe Uses of Cortisone. IL. Thomas, 1981.

Kenny, AM, et al. Effects of transdermal testosterone on bone and muscle in older men with low bioavailable testosterone levels. *J Gerontol A Biol Sci Med Sci.* 2001;56(5)266-272.

Labrie, F, et al. Effect of 12 moth dehydroepiandrosterone replacement therapy on bone, vagina and endometrium in postmenopausal women. *J Clin Endocrinol Metab.* 1997; 82(10): 3498-3505.

Lemon, HM. Estriol Prevention of Mammary Carcinoma induced by 7,12-dimethylbenzanthracene procarbazine. *Cancer Research.* 1975: 1341-1353.

Negata, C, et al. Association of dehydroepiandrosterone sulfate with serum HDL cholesterol concentrations in post-menopausal Japanese women. *Maturitas.* 1998; 31(1): 21-27.

Physicians' Desk Reference. NJ. Medical Economics Data; 1993: 856-857

Richards, DH. A post hysterectomy syndrome. *Lancet*. Oct 26, 1974: 983-984.

Rothenberg, R, Hart, K. Hormone Optimization in Preventative/Regenerative Medicine. Panda Press. CA.

Smith, YR, et al. Long term estrogen replacement is associated with improved nonverbal memory and attentional measures in postmenopausal women. *Fertil Steril*. 2001; 76(6): 1101-1107.

Tremollieres, FA, et al. Effect of Hormone Replacement therapy on age-related increase in carotid artery intima-media thickness in postmenopausal women. *Atherosclerosis*: 2000; 153(1): 81-88.

Walsh, BA, et al. 17beta-estradiol reduces tumor necrosis factor alpha-mediated LDL accumulation in the artery wall. *J Lipid Res*. 1999: 40(3): 387-96.

Wang, C, et al. Transdermal testosterone gel improves sexual function, mood, muscle strength, and body composition parameters in hypogonadal men. *J Clin Endocrinol Metab*. 2000; 85(8): 2839-2853.

Wilson, J. *Adrenal Fatigue the 21st Century Stress Syndrome*. CA. Smart Publications. 2001.

Index